A DENTAL PRACTITIONER HANDBOOK
SERIES EDITED BY DONALD D. DERRICK, D.D.S., L.D.S. R.C.S.

SILVER AMALGAM IN CLINICAL PRACTICE

I. D. GAINSFORD

B.D.S.(LOND.), F.D.S.R.C.S.(ENG.), D.D.S.HONS.(TORONTO)

*Senior Lecturer, King's College Hospital Dental School,
University of London;
Honorary Consultant, King's College Hospital*

SECOND EDITION

BRISTOL: JOHN WRIGHT & SONS LTD
1976

First edition, 1965
Second edition, 1976

ISBN 0 7236 0372 3

PRINTED IN GREAT BRITAIN BY HENRY LING LTD, A SUBSIDIARY OF JOHN WRIGHT & SONS LTD, AT THE DORSET PRESS, DORCHESTER

PREFACE TO SECOND EDITION

NOTWITHSTANDING the great strides made in recent years in the field of polymeric and glass ionomer cement filling materials, silver amalgam is still the most commonly used restorative material. There has been much research relating to silver amalgam as a restorative material which has necessitated a review of this handbook. However, it still remains clear that adherence to the well established methods of cavity preparation and amalgam manipulation is of greater importance in influencing the life of the restoration than the reliance on any marginal improvement in the physical properties claimed for the currently marketed amalgam alloys.

No attempt has been made to include in this edition the chemico-metallurgical aspects of silver amalgam alloys, for which the reader is referred to standard textbooks on dental materials. The text has been reviewed to include more recent thought in the various clinical aspects of restoring teeth with silver amalgam and to try to redress the errors and omissions found in the first edition.

The section on auxiliary retention is enlarged to include the current techniques used in this procedure as are those dealing with the choice of alloy and mercury hazards.

I would again record my thanks to the many research workers both named and unnamed in the text whose contributions to this field of dentistry have been freely consulted.

I would also acknowledge my thanks to Professor I. Curson of King's College Hospital Dental School and to Mr J. R. Grundy of the Birmingham Dental School whose help with this edition has been invaluable. In addition I would thank Mr E. W. Blewitt and the photographic department of King's College Hospital for their help with the additional photographs in this edition.

The contribution by my wife both generally with encouragement and help in all aspects associated with this handbook and specifically with all the line diagrams is gratefully acknowledged.

Finally, I again thank Mr D. Derrick, the Editor of this series, and Mr D. Emerson of John Wright & Sons Ltd, the publishers, for their forbearance and help with this second edition.

I. D. G.

PREFACE TO FIRST EDITION

THERE can be no doubt that silver amalgam is the most commonly used restorative material today, and that it has saved more teeth than any other material.

Mosteller (1957) reminds us that amalgam restorations are very rarely as bad as they look—or for that matter are inlays as good as they look. Nevertheless, there are numerous factors which influence the life of amalgam restorations, and a knowledge of these factors is essential to provide the maximum service from the restoration.

Routine examinations show that amalgam fillings can become faulty, and that failures most commonly appear as recurrent caries around the restoration, or the contour of the filling no longer assists in keeping the supporting tissue healthy.

Analyses of the causes of failure of amalgam restorations have been done by Roper (1947), Healey and Phillips (1949), and Moss (1953), who have shown that the vast majority of failures can be attributed to faulty cavity preparation or improper manipulation of the alloy. Their work stresses that the successful restoration of teeth with silver amalgam rests in the hands of the dental practitioner.

The fundamental principles of cavity preparation which were established by G. V. Black over half a century ago, and have had little modification since, were based principally on a knowledge at that time of the pathology of dental caries. It is the purpose of this handbook, while maintaining the framework of these established principles, to discuss the techniques of restoring teeth with silver amalgam, taking into consideration recent research in dental histology, histopathology, periodontology, and dental materials.

Many references have been given, not only to acknowledge the tremendous debt the clinician owes to the research worker, but also to enable the practitioner and student to delve more deeply into the subject which, owing to the concise nature of this book, has not always been possible.

I would like to thank the many research workers both named and unnamed in the text whose contributions have added enormously to our knowledge in this field of dentistry.

I would also like to thank Mr N. Livingstone Ward, of the London Hospital Dental School, and Mr J. R. Grundy, of the Birmingham Dental School, who read through the text and made many helpful suggestions which have been incorporated in this handbook. In addition my thanks are due to Mr P. Broadbery and the photographic department of the London Hospital for their help with all the photographs.

Finally I would like to express my appreciation to Mr D. Derrick, the Editor of this series, and to Mr L. G. Owens, of John Wright & Sons Ltd, the publishers, for their help and patience in the fruition of this handbook.

I. D. G.

CONTENTS

CHAPTER 1

HISTORICAL BACKGROUND

A REVIEW of the early literature in relation to the practice of dental surgery shows that silver amalgam has been in use as a dental restorative material from the beginning of the nineteenth century, and that for many years it was considered a sort of Cinderella among dental fillings. The early amalgams were made by mixing with mercury the filings from Spanish or Mexican silver coins, since these coins had a high silver content. This produced a harsh mass which was difficult to mix; it hardened very slowly and expanded enormously, and also stained the teeth black. It is little wonder that with these qualities it should have failed so utterly, and it was these early experiences which resulted in the slow establishment of amalgam as a reputable restorative material.

The first dental silver amalgam is supposed to have been introduced into England by Bell in 1819, and was known as 'Bell's putty'. Its introduction to the North American continent in 1833, under the much more salubrious name of the 'Royal Mineral Succedaneum', is attributed to the Cawcour brothers. These practitioners, by successful advertising and speedy, slovenly work, succeeded in establishing a fortune for themselves and a name of ill-repute for amalgam.

The failure of amalgam in its early use, or more accurately its early abuse, was so formidable that in 1843 a resolution was passed by the American Society of Dental Surgeons, the first organized dental society in the U.S.A., declaring the use of amalgam a 'malpractice'. Thus the 'Amalgam War' began. In 1845 the 'Amalgam Pledge' was also adopted by the same society, which consisted of all members signing a pledge not to use amalgam; those refusing to sign were expelled. This pledge was rescinded in 1850, officially ending the amalgam war. Nevertheless, many practitioners after this time considered amalgam a complete failure in its application to dentistry.

A great number of individuals and institutions have been responsible for research into silver amalgam. The first of these research programmes was conducted by John Tomes in 1861 (*Trans. Odontol. Soc. G.B.*, vol. III), who measured shrinkage of a number of amalgams. In 1871 Charles Tomes measured shrinkage and expansion by specific-gravity tests, and in 1874 Thomas B. Hitchcock (*Trans. N.Y. Odontol. Soc.*) did some important work in measuring

1

more accurately, by means of a micrometer, changes of amalgam form.

However, it was not until the classic work of G. V. Black in 1896 that a systematic study was made of the properties and manner of manipulation of silver amalgam and its relation to cavity preparation. As a result, some of the more important failures associated with the earlier amalgams were overcome. It is interesting to note that, although great strides have been made in dental research since G. V. Black, many of his suggested techniques for amalgam restorations are generally accepted today. In fact new methods are often described as variations or modifications of those used by Black.

In 1930 a dental survey organized by the American Dental Association Research Commission showed that only a few of the proprietary amalgam alloys on the market and tested by the National Bureau of Standards were really reliable, and this resulted in the production of the American Dental Association's Specification No. 1 for amalgam. Since then there has been a revision of this specification in 1934, in 1960 and again in 1970. The main differences between the 1970 A.D.A. Specification No. 1 for amalgam and the previous specifications are the inclusion of a diametral tensile test as an indication of the rate of hardening of the amalgam as distinct from a compressive strength test; and adjustments in the setting change and flow requirements that are due to changes in test procedures. This latter factor is necessitated by the change from hand trituration to mechanical mixing. The British Standards Institution provided a specification for amalgam in 1957 and again in 1961 and this is currently under review. At the present time there is a great variety of amalgam alloys which complies with these specifications.

CHAPTER 2

CAVITY PREPARATION

THE main drawback of silver amalgam fillings from the patient's point of view is the fact that they tarnish and occasionally corrode in the mouth, and are thus generally unsightly. It is for this reason that they are confined to the posterior teeth, and therefore only the principles of cavity preparation involving those types of cavities which are normally restored with amalgam will be discussed.

The object of cavity preparation is the mechanical removal of caries and the leaving of the remaining tooth tissue in such a way that, after restoration, it will be able:

1. To prevent the subsequent recurrence of caries in that area of the tooth;
2. To withstand masticatory forces;
3. To assume a more ideal anatomic form.

G. V. Black has described six stages in the preparation of a cavity, and, although after having completed each stage it will be found that certain aspects of the subsequent stages will have been fulfilled, it is still a good maxim to complete each stage as perfectly as possible before proceeding to the next one.

The stages in order of sequence are enumerated below, and an attempt will be made to discuss the more important aspects in each case:

1. Establish the outline form.
2. Obtain resistance and retention form.
3. Remove carious dentine.
4. Obtain convenience form.
5. Finish the enamel walls and margins.
6. Perform the toilet of the cavity.

1. THE OUTLINE FORM

The principle of establishing outline form means the cutting of the cavity to the outline it will have when the cavity has been prepared. Thus the design of the cavity is established at the outset.

In order to achieve this outline form, two factors have to be considered: (*a*) removal of caries at the amelo-dentinal junction; (*b*) extension for prevention.

Removal of Caries at the Amelo-dentinal Junction
Although there is no complete agreement as to the method of caries

3

penetration of enamel, all authorities agree that, once the amelo-dentinal junction has been reached, the rate of spread of the caries is much more rapid, and that the most marked spread is in a lateral direction underneath the enamel (*Fig.* 1). Furthermore, it is agreed that the enamel prisms are at their weakest and most likely to fracture when they are unsupported by sound dentine.

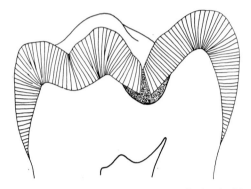

Fig. 1. Lateral spread of caries below the amelo-dentinal junction.

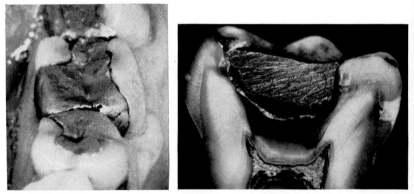

Fig. 2. 'Ditched' amalgam restorations.

Fig. 3. Amalgam filling surrounded by recurrent caries.

It is therefore essential to remove all enamel undermined by caries or left undermined as a result of the removal of that caries at the amelo-dentinal junction area. This will prevent the restoration failing as a result of subsequent fracture of unsupported enamel at the periphery of the filling, producing the classic 'ditched amalgam' (*Fig.* 2), or the filling finishing up in a 'sea of caries' (*Fig.* 3), following either recurrent caries occurring in this ditched margin or being the result of caries left from the original lesion.

4

When removing caries under cusps, it is often found that it is only when the overhanging enamel is removed that one can reveal the presence of more caries in the amelo-dentinal junction. If the removal of this caries results in the enamel forming the cusp becoming

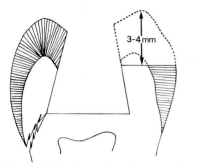

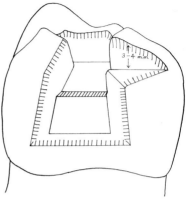

Fig. 4. Reduction of weak cusp to prevent its subsequent fracture. Note that sufficient must be removed to provide adequate thickness of amalgam reforming cusp.

Fig. 5. Reduction of part of cusp.

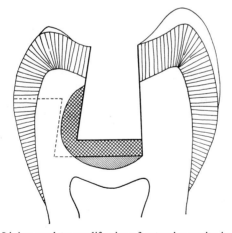

Fig. 6. Lining used to modify size of extensive cavity in order to reduce bulk of amalgam, the thermal expansion of which could lead to fracture of cusp. Dotted line indicates outline form for stronger restoration. Note need for non-irritant sub-base in deep cavities.

unsupported, it will often become necessary to cut back the cusp. Provided the tooth is still to be restored with amalgam, enough tooth tissue must be removed to give a vertical height of at least 3 mm of amalgam, so as to ensure that there is adequate bulk of

5

filling reforming the cusp which is able to withstand masticatory forces without fracturing (*Fig.* 4).

There would, of course, be modifications if only part of the cusp is involved (*Fig.* 5). The clinical judgement of the operator is then needed to decide if the remaining tooth tissue will withstand occlusal stresses and, if not, whether it is wiser to relieve the occlusal stress by grinding the opposing tooth rather than extend the cavity to include the whole cusp. The retention of a cusp can sometimes be maintained by filling the undermined areas with zinc phosphate cement (*Fig.* 6); in order to avoid the risk of fracture resulting from thermal expansion of an excessive bulk of amalgam. However, if such a supported cusp is subjected to heavy mastication, it is unlikely to be retained for long. The removal of caries at the amelo-dentinal junction is best achieved with a round burr, and the

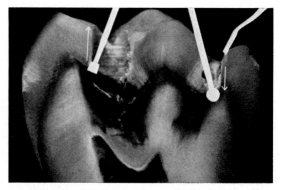

Fig. 7. Removal of caries at the amelo-dentinal junction and undermined enamel.

subsequent removal of undermined enamel with chisels (*Fig.* 7). Another satisfactory technique is to use an inverted cone burr placed in the dentine just below the amelo-dentinal junction, and while revolving to pull occlusally (*Fig.* 7). The advantage of this technique is that there is no risk of exposing the pulp while the amelo-dentinal caries and the overhanging enamel are removed with the burr.

Extension for Prevention
It has been established that certain areas of the tooth surface are more susceptible to caries, either because of being in areas where food can easily stagnate or because of the presence of natural pits and fissures which provide nidi for the cariogenic processes. It is for this reason that it is a general procedure to include in the cavity

outline wherever possible those areas of the tooth which have a predisposition to future decay, and which are in close proximity to the original carious lesion. Black (1947) termed this procedure 'extension for prevention', while McGehee et al. (1956) called it 'cutting for immunity'.

However, it should be remembered that such factors as age, susceptibility to caries, relative position of the gingiva, alignment of teeth, standard of oral hygiene and the general health of the patient must be borne in mind when deciding how radical the extension for prevention should be. Only in cases of gross caries susceptibility is the more radical extension advisable.

Outline Form in Class I Cavities

In pit and fissure cavities the outline will be formed by first removing the cariously undermined enamel, and then following all the fissures which lead into the carious area. These fissures are removed until the cavity margin is bounded by a smooth outline of enamel supported by dentine. If two pit or fissure cavities are in close proximity, as is commonly seen in upper molar teeth where the mesial and distal pits are separated by an oblique ridge, or the lower first

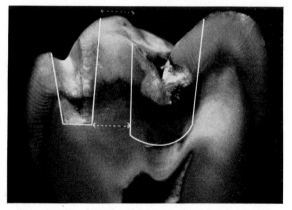

Fig. 8. Outline form justifying retention of oblique ridge.

premolar where a transverse ridge separates mesial and distal pits, the clinical judgement of the operator is needed to decide whether the cavities should be joined. This decision, of course, will be based on whether the remaining bridge of enamel is strong enough to withstand fracture (*Figs.* 8–10). It is wise to prepare each cavity separately at the same appointment, and then see if there is an adequate bridge of dentine-supported enamel. Care should be taken to make the walls on either side of the oblique or transverse ridge occlusally convergent. This will provide the separating ridge with a wide base, and so increase its strength (*Figs.* 8–10).

McGehee et al. (1956) consider that deep developmental grooves should also be removed in extension for prevention. However, since this procedure may seriously weaken the remaining tooth structure, this should only be followed in the very caries susceptible patient. De Boer (1956) and many others support this concept, that only in cases of extreme caries susceptibility is such radical extension permissible. Pearson (1959) suggests that, where the fissures approach the buccal and lingual surfaces of the tooth, or extend well into the marginal ridges, the burr should be inclined so as to cut out the defect in the enamel without removing the non-carious underlying dentine (*Fig.* 11). In this way the marginal walls of the

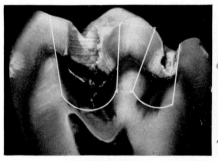
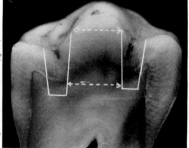

Fig. 9. Outline form requiring removal of oblique ridge.

Fig. 10. Outline form justifying retention of transverse ridge.

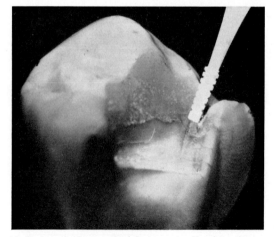

Fig. 11. Removal of a terminal fissure extending into the marginal ridge using a 700 tapered fissure burr.

cavity are not unnecessarily weakened. It should be remembered that outline form is also influenced by a desire to keep the margins of the cavity away from heavy biting areas wherever possible, in view of the inherent weakness of amalgam.

Although the most common site for these Class I pit and fissure cavities is on the occlusal surfaces of premolar and molar teeth, often they also occur on the buccal surfaces of lower molars and on the palatal surfaces of upper incisors. In addition, they occur, though less frequently, on the palatal aspect of upper molars, either where they are an extension of the distal-occlusal fissure, or in the fissure formed by the additional palatal cusp or tubercle of Carabelli. Frequently it is possible to limit the extension of these cavities to the single surface they involve. However, if it is not possible to ensure that a smooth periphery to the cavity can be obtained, then the cavity must be extended on to the occlusal surface, and the fissures are cut out as in a routine occlusal cavity.

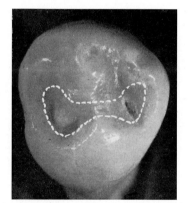

Fig. 12. Contour of cavity outline to provide maximum strength to cusp and marginal ridges.

Thus it can be seen that the outline form in pit and fissure caries will be controlled not only by the extent of the caries, but also by the anatomic form of the tooth's surface in which the cavity is being cut. The walls around the cusps are cut in sweeping curves to prevent pulpal exposure and maintain the maximum strength of the cusp, and the mesial and distal walls are cut parallel to the direction of the mesial and distal contour of the tooth respectively (*Fig.* 12).

Outline Form in Class II Cavities

Class II cavities are either the result of the decay of interproximal smooth surfaces, which usually starts at or slightly gingival to the contact area, or are the result of an extension from a pit or fissure

9

lesion. This extension of a Class I cavity into a Class II cavity may be due, in addition to the spread of the original Class I carious lesion, to the removal of too much marginal ridge tissue, having in mind the need for ensuring adequate strength of the marginal ridge.

In order to gain access to the interproximal caries, so as to fulfil the principles of removal of caries at the amelo-dentinal junction, and also extension for prevention, it is necessary to involve the occlusal surface.

There are, however, a few exceptions to the need to involve the occlusal surface, and these are:

a. Where the approximal tooth is missing and access to the carious lesion is possible without involving the occlusal surface (*Fig.* 13). An interproximal space of less than 1 unit usually makes access difficult, and the classic Class II approach via the occlusal surface is easier. It should be noted that when the missing tooth is

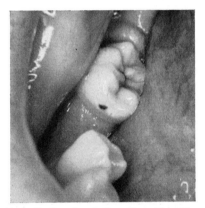

Fig. 13. Indication for single surface Class II cavity.

to be replaced by an artificial tooth, fixed or removable, the patient should be given specific instructions on cleaning the amalgam enamel junction. This will avoid the need to extend the cavity on to the occlusal surface in order to take the periphery of the cavity to self-cleansing areas.

b. Where the decay is exclusively in cementum and it is possible to have adequate access to remove all the caries and make the cavity sufficiently retentive for the amalgam filling.

c. As a temporary procedure.

In these circumstances, a single surface cavity is prepared, and the outline is formed by the removal of caries at the amelo-dentinal and cemento-dentinal junctions. If the extension of the cavity occlusally

10

in any way jeopardizes the strength of the marginal ridge, then the cavity should be extended on to the occlusal surface.

The points of special interest concerning the outline form of a Class II amalgam cavity are best considered under three headings: (*a*) Position of the gingival margin; (*b*) Position of the embrasure walls; (*c*) Position of the occlusal dovetail.

a. THE POSITION OF THE GINGIVAL MARGIN: Research work by Zander (1957), Waerhaug (1960), and App (1961) has modified our ideas on whether the gingival floor should be placed above, below, or at the level of the crest of the gingival margin.

These workers have established that restorations in amalgam, as well as acrylic and silicate cement, do produce chronic inflammation of the gingival tissue. The tissue response is similar to that of tissue response to calculus (*Fig.* 14).

App prepared 36 buccal Class V cavities in a young dog's teeth, using a No. 558 carbide fissure burr, with the cavities extending below the crest of the gingival tissue. Twelve cavities were filled with silicate cement, 12 with amalgam, and 12 with cast gold inlays. In the case of the amalgam cavities, the amalgam was contoured immediately after insertion, and all excess amalgam was carefully removed. Twenty-four hours later the restorations were polished with Burlew's discs and also with tin oxide in a rubber cup.

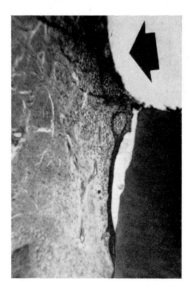

Fig. 14. Section of tooth and adjacent gingival tissue where gingival margin of cavity is placed in the gingival sulcus (*by courtesy of J. Waerhaug*). Arrow indicates chronic inflammation against amalgam restoration.

11

Although the clinical appearance of the gingival tissue subsequent to the completion of these restorations was normal, the histological examination after 7 and 30 days showed marked inflammation of the gingival tissue. The control side consisted of the lingual aspect of these teeth having a simulated amount of instrumentation for an equivalent period of cavity preparation time by using a No. 558 fissure burr with the terminal blades removed. The results on the control side showed few inflammatory cells and no epithelial proliferation.

App's major point is that 'since calculus is an aetiological factor in periodontal disease and the sulcus epithelium responds to silicate and amalgam as it does to calculus, these restorative materials must also be considered aetiological factors in periodontal disease'.

On the other hand, Blackwell (1940) and Demajo (1954) are of the opinion that the good that can be achieved in the prevention of recurrent caries by extending the cavity into the gingival crevice far

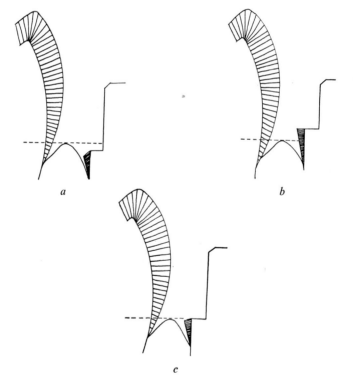

Fig. 15. Position of cavo-gingival line angle in relation to crest of gingival margin. *a*, Extension into gingival sulcus necessitated by presence of caries; *b*, Inadequate gingival extension; *c*, Ideal extension to level of crest of gingival margin.

outweighs the harm, if any, that might result to the gingivae. McCall (1926) postulated the theory that the alkali secretions in the gingival crevice tended to make this area relatively immune by neutralizing the acids present in the cariogenic process, and consequently inhibited recurrent caries. However, the consensus of recent research into this subject of gingival margin placement points to finishing the cavo-gingival line angle at the crest of the gingival margin (*Fig.* 15), and that the encouragement of the patient in maintaining a high standard of oral hygiene will prevent the occurrence of secondary caries in this area.

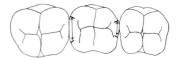

Fig. 16. Effect of contour on buccolingual extension of embrasure walls.

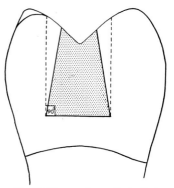

Fig. 18. Converging walls to the box provide: *a*, Conservation of tooth tissue; *b*, Retention form; *c*, Less occlusal stress on restoration; *d*, Greater cusp strength; *e*, Improved aesthetics.

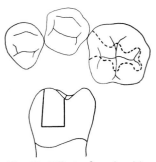

Fig. 17. Effect of malposition of contact area on location of proximal box.

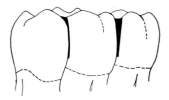

Fig. 19. Effect of angle of embrasure wall on aesthetic appearance of restoration. More amalgam is visible in distal restoration where buccogingival line angle is 90°.

If caries, either as obvious caries or as a hypocalcified white line, extends below the level of the gingival crest, the cavity must be extended to include this caries, but in the vast majority of cases of interproximal caries where this is not so, the cavo-gingival line angle should not be extended below the crest of the gingiva.

b. THE POSITION OF THE EMBRASURE WALLS: In obtaining adequate extension for prevention, the position of the proximal buccal and lingual cavo-surface line angles is governed by:

13

i. The natural contour of the tooth in a buccolingual direction; the greater the convexity of the proximal surface of the tooth, the less the extension is required to get the margins in a self-cleansing area (*Fig.* 16).

ii. The relationship of the tooth to its neighbour (*Fig.* 17).

Simon (1951) suggests that the extension of the proximal cavity into the embrasures is sufficient if the point of a right-angle probe, when placed in the buccogingivo-axial and linguogingivo-axial point angles, can pass freely between the margins of the cavity and the adjacent tooth. The criterion, however, for achieving adequate extension buccally and lingually is that the bristles of a toothbrush must be able to keep the amalgam enamel junction clean.

Markley's (1951) technique, which he has shown on plaster models, for illustrating the proximal outline form is to hold a flat pencil against the adjacent tooth with the lead touching the tooth to be restored, so describing the proximal cavity outline. This will result in the buccal and lingual margins being approximately parallel respectively to the buccal and lingual contours of the adjacent tooth.

The advantages of having the proximal lingual and buccal walls converging in an occlusal direction (*Fig.* 18) are that it:

α. Requires less removal of tooth tissue.

β. Assists in the retention of the restoration from displacement in an occlusal direction.

γ. Presents less of the restoration to occlusal stress. If the buccal and lingual walls were parallel, as suggested by Black, then the buccolingual width of the proximo-occlusal part of the restoration would be governed by the minimum buccolingual width required to make all parts of the proximal box self-cleansing. Converging walls, the cavo-surface line angles of which are still in self-cleansing areas, result in a narrower buccolingual width to the occlusal surface of the box. This results in the box being subjected to less occlusal stress than if the walls of the box had been parallel. Nadal et al. (1961) have shown that, by reducing the occlusal stress on an amalgam restoration, there is less likelihood of fracture of the restoration, even if a weaker, high residual-mercury-content amalgam is used.

δ. Provides greater cusp strength. Vale (1959) has shown that when the width of the isthmus of the cavity is increased beyond a quarter of the intercuspal distance, the resistance of the cusp to fracture is greatly weakened.

ε. Improves aesthetics. Bronner (1931) originally made the point that, by converging the walls of a proximal cavity, less amalgam was visible (*Fig.* 19) while the principle of extension for prevention was still observed.

Studies by Mahler (1958), Guard et al. (1958), with photo-elastic stress analyses of amalgam restorations, have shown that rounded cavity line angles produce less stress concentrations in the amalgam than do sharp angles. Although this will be discussed more fully under 'Resistance Form', it should be pointed out that they recommend that the buccogingival and linguogingival angles should be rounded (*see Fig.* 30).

While discussing the embrasure walls of a proximal cavity, the correct angle formed by the buccal and lingual walls at their cavo-surface line angles should also be noted. In order to obtain maximum strength for the amalgam and enamel, the proximal buccal and lingual walls should form a right angle with the tooth surface (*Fig.* 20).

Ultra high-speed cutting instruments result all too commonly in a flaring of the embrasure walls (*Fig.* 21). The effect of flaring these walls is that it is difficult to ensure adequate condensation of amalgam into the narrow angles formed by these flared walls and the matrix band. In addition, the weak spur of amalgam which results is very prone to fracture.

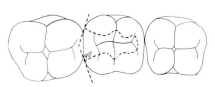

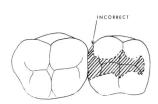

| *Fig.* 20. Embrasure walls should form a right angle at cavity margin. | *Fig.* 21. Flaring of embrasure wall leads to a weak restoration. |

c. THE POSITION OF THE OCCLUSAL DOVETAIL: Occlusally, the outline form of a Class II cavity includes the pits and fissures as in a Class I cavity previously described, in order to obtain 'extension for prevention'. However, in addition to removing pits and fissures, adequate provision must be made for widening that part of the occlusal cavity farthest away from the proximal box, so as to provide a dovetail or lock (*Fig.* 22). The function of the lock is to prevent displacement of the restoration in the direction of the missing wall.

Outline Form in Class V Cavities

Class V cavities are smooth surface cavities located at the gingival third of buccal and, more rarely, lingual surfaces of teeth. At first the defect may appear as a whitish chalky line close to the gingival margin. If this area is kept clean and polished, then the need for the preparation of a cavity may be prevented.

If, however, there is enough caries penetration of the enamel or cementum for a probe to catch in it, a cavity will have to be prepared.

15

Markley (1955) points out that the threat of recurrent caries is greater in gingival third regions than in any other site. It is for this reason that special care must be taken to ensure that the outline of this cavity includes the stagnation areas prone to decay, and that careful instruction in maintaining efficient oral hygiene is given to the patient.

The outline of a Class V cavity should extend:

a. Mesially and distally to the proximal angles of the tooth (*Fig.* 23), since these areas are considered less susceptible to decay (McGehee et al., 1956, *Fig.* 24).

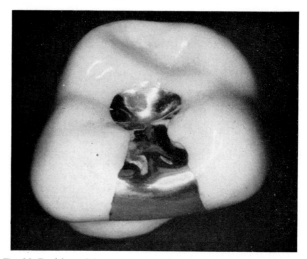

Fig. 22. Position of dovetail to assist in retention of the restoration.

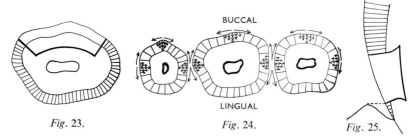

Fig. 23.   *Fig.* 24.   *Fig.* 25.

Fig. 23. Mesial and distal extension of Class V.

Fig. 24. Areas prone to decay on circumference of posterior teeth. Lingual surface and buccal embrasure angles are relatively immune. (*After McGehee.*)

Fig. 25. Gingival extension of Class V cavity to level of the crest of the gingival margin.

b. Gingivally to the crest of the gingival margin, in order to minimize gingival irritation (*Fig.* 25). If caries extends subgingivally, then the cavity must be extended to include this caries; and conversely, if there is limited caries and gingival recession, then the cavity would not be extended to the gingival margin.

c. Occlusally to sound tooth tissue. It should be carried far enough occlusally to allow the cleansing action of cheek movements and tooth-brushing to keep the enamel–amalgam junction clean.

There are two schools of thought concerning the outline form of the occlusal margin (*Fig.* 26):

i. The traditional kidney shape, which is more conservative of tissue.

ii. The Ferrier Class V cavity, originally designed for gold foil restorations, was recommended by Markley (1955) for Class V cavities to be restored with amalgam. Here the occlusal and gingival margins are cut parallel to the occlusal surface of the tooth. Extension beyond the mesial and distal margins of the tooth are carried as projections from the main body of the preparation.

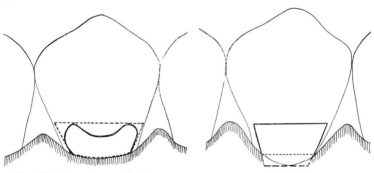

Fig. 26. Comparison of Class V outline forms. Dotted line represents Ferrier outline form.

Fig. 27. Disadvantage of horizontal gingival outline form to Class V cavity.

Ferrier (1959) agrees that in some instances, for example at the cervix of upper incisors where there is a marked gingival curvature, it is not possible to have a horizontal gingival wall. In this instance, if the gingival wall were to remain horizontal, it would be necessary to cut considerably below the gingival margin mesially and distally, or have the middle part of the gingival wall not subgingival at all (*Fig.* 27). He suggests that, where there is marked gingival curvature, the gingival wall is also curved, but the occlusal wall still remains horizontal. This would also apply to marked gingival curvature in premolar teeth.

17

Markley (1955) considers that the justification for using the Ferrier type of outline form for amalgam restorations is the improved aesthetics when there are several Class V cavities present, as they tend to blend more easily. It is questionable if the improvement in aesthetics justifies this less conservative approach to Class V cavity preparations (*Fig.* 28).

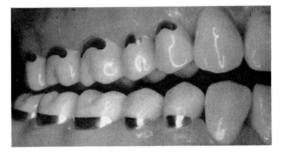

Fig. 28. Comparison of aesthetic appearance of Class V outline forms.

2. RESISTANCE AND RETENTION FORM

Since both these requirements are generally attained by the same technical procedures, they will be discussed together in their application to cavities to be restored with amalgam. They are, however, two distinct factors.

Resistance Form
Resistance form is the ability of the restoration to withstand applied stresses. In deciding on the resistance form of a restoration, one must also consider the resistance form of the remaining tooth tissue. The prepared tooth must be able to withstand, without fracturing, adequate packing pressures to produce a properly condensed filling, in addition to masticatory stresses. Amalgam should only be used in those cavities where the restoration can be supported and retained by the tooth tissue, and not where the restoration is primarily intended to support the tooth unless, however, auxiliary retention is employed.

Since silver amalgam resists compressive forces far better than shear or tension forces, the cavity should be designed to receive compressive forces. Consequently, the cavity is cut at right angles to the occlusal plane, with the pulpal and gingival floors being horizontal. Work done by Mahler (1958) and Guard et al. (1958) on photo-elastic stress analyses of amalgam have tended to alter previously held concepts that the pulpal and gingival floors

18

should be flat and that all internal line angles should be sharp. These workers have shown that gently rounded pulpal or gingival floors and gently rounded internal line angles show the best distribution of stress in the amalgam restoration.

It has previously been recognized that it was only the axiopulpal line angle that was to be rounded or bevelled. The reason for this was to increase the bulk of amalgam in an area where there was a change of direction of the restoration (*Fig.* 29). This applies equally to the axiopulpal line angles in Class II restorations, and to that in the buccal or lingual extensions from the occlusal cavity. The justification for bevelling the axiopulpal line angles has been endorsed by the results of the photo-elastic stress analyses, where a sharp angle shows marked stress concentrations in amalgam, which will result, it is reasoned, in a weaker restoration. However, the clinical importance of rounding all the other internal line angles is doubtful, since properly condensed amalgam restorations are unlikely to fracture at these points. Unless the round-ended, flat fissure burr seen in *Fig.* 30 is used, it is difficult to achieve rounded angles without further undercutting the walls of the cavity.

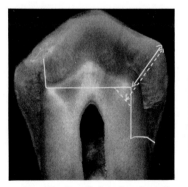

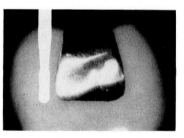

Fig. 29. Bevelled axiopulpal line angle to provide additional bulk of restorative material.

Fig. 30. The use of round-ended fissure burrs to provide rounded cavity angles.

The axial wall should be cut parallel to the long axis of the tooth, just on the dentine side of the amelo-dentinal junction (*Fig.* 31), unless caries dictates further penetration. However, if the gingival floor has to be taken below the amelo-cemental junction, the angulation of the axial wall will have to be changed, and made to run parallel to the contour of the proximal surface of the tooth involved (*Fig.* 32). It is essential to ensure that there is adequate gingival floor to support the proximal box. If in deep proximal boxes the axial wall is cut parallel to the long axis of the tooth, it will either result in possible exposure of the pulp, or insufficient gingival floor to provide adequate resistance form to compressive forces.

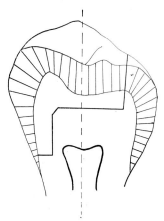

Fig. 31. Axial wall cut parallel to long axis of tooth.

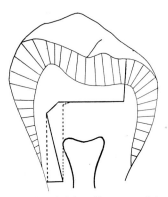

Fig. 32. Axial wall cut parallel to proximal contour of tooth. This will avoid exposure of pulp or insufficient gingival floor in deep proximal box.

Retention Form

Obtaining retention form may be defined as producing a cavity whereby the restoration can withstand displacing forces.

These displacing forces are of two kinds: (*a*) the component forces of mastication; (*b*) the pull of sticky food.

G. V. Black recommended that the walls of a cavity should be cut at right angles to the pulpal floor, and that slight undercuts should be cut in the dentine to retain the amalgam restoration. Although the exact direction of the enamel prisms at the surface of a tooth is variable, all authorities agree that the general direction of the prisms is approximately at right angles to any given surface of the tooth's circumference. It is for this reason that, in preparing the walls of a cavity, an attempt is made to have the walls at near right angles to the tooth's surface, and not necesssarily at right angles to the pulpal floor. In this way the maximum edge strength of the enamel and amalgam is maintained.

In the mechanically correct cavity of *Fig.* 33 it will be seen that the walls of the cavity are at right angles to the pulpal floor as well as to the tooth's surface, and retention is obtained by cutting undercuts in the dentine below the amelo-dentinal junction. However, this type of cavity would only be seen in the completely flattened occlusal surface, or possibly in a small Class V cavity.

Kornfield (1952) has pointed out that tooth surfaces consist of inclined planes and the effect of parallel walls to a cavity in such a tooth would be to increase the strength of the enamel edge enormously but this would be at the expense of the amalgam restoration (*Fig.* 34). Kornfield suggests that if the walls are cut at right angles to the tooth's surface, they will produce adequate retention, while at the same time providing the butt joint between amalgam and enamel (*Fig.* 35). This also results in reducing the occlusal stress taken by the restoration by reducing the occlusal width of the cavity relative to the width of the base.

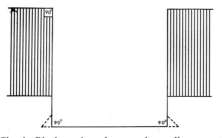

Fig. 33. Classic Black cavity where cavity walls are cut at right angles to pulpal floor, providing maximum edge strength for enamel and amalgam.

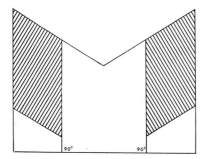

Fig. 34. Parallel walls in cuspal areas result in weak edge for amalgam restoration.

However, Simon (1956) has suggested a slight modification whereby the enamel prisms are further protected. Instead of a right angle at the cavo-surface line angle, an angle of 100° is produced which will result in the terminal ends of the enamel prisms being cut across (*Fig.* 36). Simon calls this a 'full bevel', since the full depth of the enamel wall is cut at this inclination, unlike the 'short bevel' in gold restorations, where a cavo-surface line angle of 135°

21

is produced and only extended up to half way through the depth of the enamel.

A 100° cavo-surface line angle will result in the amalgam having an 80° angle if the previous contour of the cusp is reproduced. Since this angle is produced through the whole depth of the amalgam restoration, it is doubtful whether the amalgam will be significantly weakened. Nevertheless, by modifying the inclination of the carved surface of the restoration from the enamel margin of the cavity, the amalgam angle can also be increased, so enhancing the edge strength of the restoration (*Fig.* 36). It may be necessary to allow for the increased thickness of amalgam by occlusal adjustment of an opposing high point of enamel.

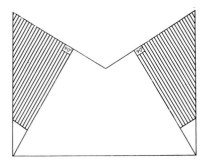

Fig. 35. Cavity walls cut at right angles to tooth surface.

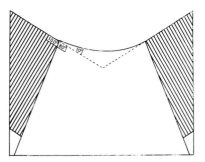

Fig. 36. Enamel angle increased to provide added enamel edge strength and 'full bevel'. Amalgam surface is raised to increase amalgam edge strength.

The additional advantage of increasing the cavo-surface line angle above 90° is especially seen in high cusped teeth where extension of a wall producing a 90° cavo-surface line angle into dentine could seriously undermine the cusp (*Fig.* 37).

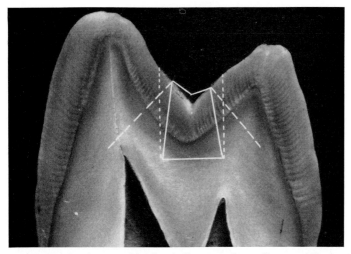

Fig. 37. Continuous white line indicates cavity outline providing retention form and satisfactory edge strength for enamel and amalgam. Parallel dotted lines will result in weak amalgam edge. Convergent dotted lines can weaken cusps or lead to pulpal exposure.

Resistance and Retention Form in Class I Cavities

In Class I cavities the pulpal floor is cut to below the amelo-dentinal junction, in order to ensure the removal of all caries at the amelo-dentinal junction and also to provide adequate depth for retention of the filling. Gabel (1957) suggests that the depth of the cavity in sound dentine should be about 1 mm beyond the amelo-dentinal junction. The cavity should not be deepened beyond this for

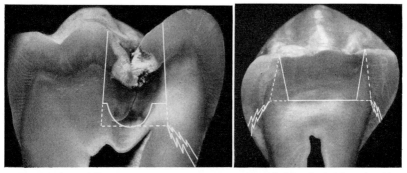

Fig. 38. Dotted line represents unnecessary deepening of pulpal floor, which can lead to fracture of cusp.

Fig. 39. Marginal ridges should not be undermined.

23

increased retention, since the deeper the preparation the greater the pulpal injury. Markley (1951), in addition, points out that excessive deepening of the pulpal floor can weaken the surrounding dentine support for the cusps (*Fig.* 38). Adequate retention is achieved by the occlusally convergent walls in the cuspal regions of the tooth only. The mesial and distal walls of the cavity at the marginal ridges should be occlusally divergent, in order to give the marginal ridges as wide a base as possible to maintain their strength, having in mind the natural constriction of the tooth below the contact areas (*Fig.* 39).

The walls bounding a transverse or oblique ridge should be occlusally convergent, since undercutting these ridges can easily lead to their subsequent breakdown (*see Figs.* 8–10).

Resistance and Retention Form in Class II Cavities

A Class II cavity is made up of two components—namely, the proximal box and the occlusal lock. Although each assists in the retention of the other, the preparation should ensure that the retention of each component can be independent. This will increase the retention of the restoration enormously, and should it be necessary to restore another surface of the tooth at a later date, it will be possible to involve the occlusal surface without weakening the existing proximal filling.

In the case of the occlusal lock the resistance and retention form is obtained by:

a. Cutting the walls of the cavity at nearly right angles to the tooth's surface, so providing convergent walls, especially in the cuspal areas. If a marginal or transverse ridge is to be left intact, the principles outlined in Class I cavities must be observed. The pulpal floor is cut into dentine to about 1 mm below the amelo-dentinal junction.

b. Cutting a dovetail or lock to prevent displacement of the occlusal restoration in the direction of the missing wall. As pointed out under the heading of 'Outline Form', this is placed away from the proximal box in a two-surface restoration, so as to prevent weakening the cusps in the region of the junction of the box and lock (*see Fig.* 22).

However, in a three-surface restoration the other box or extension provides the equivalent function of an occlusal dovetail. The anatomy of lower molar teeth facilitates the provision of a central dovetail, which greatly aids retention in M.O.D. cavities.

Similarly, the box should be independently retentive. Displacement in an occlusal direction is prevented by the occlusally convergent walls, as discussed in 'Outline Form' (*see Fig.* 18). In addition to the occlusal dovetail, retention of the box from proximal displacement is achieved by:

i. *Gingival Lock.* With the use of sharp Black's marginal trimmers or a small rose-head burr, the gingival dentine floor is slightly inclined in an apical direction from just before the amelo-dentinal junction to the axial wall (*Fig.* 40).

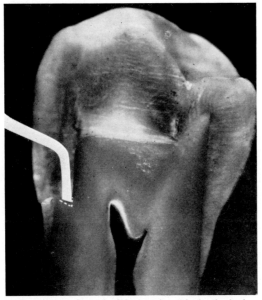

Fig. 40. Provision of gingival lock using Black gingival margin trimmer.

ii. *Embrasure Retention Grooves.* These grooves are cut in the dentine of the buccal and lingual embrasure walls of the box. They should extend occlusally up from the gingival floor to about the level of the pulpal floor (*Fig.* 41). This can best be done with a 700 tapered fissure burr (*Fig.* 42), and in order to avoid the risk of pulpal involvement the following points should be noted:

α. The direction is parallel to the amelo-dentinal junction.

β. The grooves should be progressively shallower away from gingival floor.

γ. The grooves should not extend occlusally above the level of the pulpal floor.

The foregoing principles of resistance and retention form can be applied to all Class II preparations in premolars and molars. However, in restoring Class II cavities in lower first premolars, there are additional problems related to cavity design, because of the peculiar anatomy of this tooth.

25

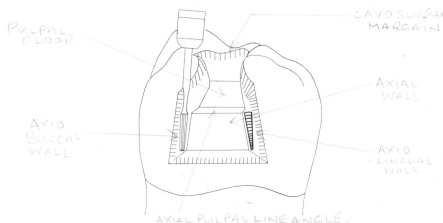

Fig. 41. Retention grooves in embrasure walls of box.

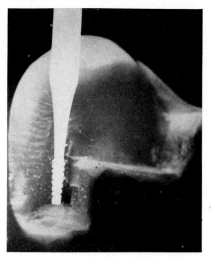

Fig. 42. Provision of retention groove using 700 tapered fissure
burr.

Class II Restorations in Mandibular First Premolars

Although this is a two-cusped tooth, it is more like a lower canine
with a lingual cusp, rather than resembling the other premolars.
The lingual cusp is very much smaller than the buccal cusp, and is
never in occlusion with its opposing tooth, unless grossly misplaced.
Sometimes a median ridge joins these two cusps, resulting in mesial
and distal pits or fossae. The pulp chamber is relatively large, with

26

a cornua extending into the buccal cusp, but seldom into the lingual cusp (*Fig.* 43).

Thus, in Class I or Class II cavities in this tooth, the preceding principles of cavity preparation for Class I and Class II cavities will have to be modified to take advantage of the knowledge of the morphology of this tooth.

Caries in either or both of the pits can often be cut out without destroying the median ridge (*see Fig.* 10). However, if this ridge has to be undermined to remove caries, then the mesial and distal pits should be joined (*see Fig.* 12).

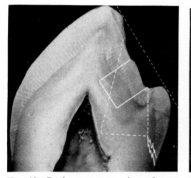 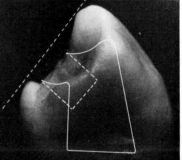

Fig. 43. Cavity cut approximately at right angles to an imaginary line joining buccal and lingual cusps of mandibular first premolar. Dotted line represents outline form that could lead to pulpal exposure and fracture of weak lingual cusp.

Fig. 44. Relation of box to lock in mandibular first premolar.

The occlusal cavity is cut at the expense of the buccal cusp, with the central fissure representing the lingual cavo-surface line angle. The cavity walls are cut approximately at right angles to an imaginary line joining the buccal and lingual cusps (*Fig.* 43). These walls are cut parallel to each other, so that the buccal cusp is not excessively undermined.

The mesial and distal extensions of the median fissure into the buccal cusp are also cut out (*see Fig.* 12).

The pulpal floor is cut parallel to the imaginary line joining the buccal and lingual cusps. This will avoid the risk of pulpal exposure, while at the same time allowing the lingual and buccal walls to finish below the amelo-dentinal junction. A pulpal floor which is horizontal and entirely in dentine can easily expose the buccal cornua of the pulp (*Fig.* 43).

The proximal box is cut at right angles to the occlusal plane of the buccal cusp (*Fig.* 44), following the general principles outlined in

27

Class II cavity preparation, and the gingival floor is cut horizontal, as previously described.

It is important to ensure that the proximal box is self-retentive, although the different paths of withdrawal of the occlusal and proximal parts of the cavity will assist in the retention of the restoration.

In a two-surface Class II restoration, the dovetail is provided by cutting into the proximal median fissure extension of the buccal cusp farthest away from the box. No extension is made into the lingual cusp.

Resistance and Retention Form in Class V Cavities

Although a Class V restoration is subjected to minimal stresses and displacing forces, provision for adequate resistance and retention form must be established.

The walls are cut parallel to the direction of the enamel prisms, so as to provide a butt joint at the cavo-surface line angle (*Figs.* 45, 46).

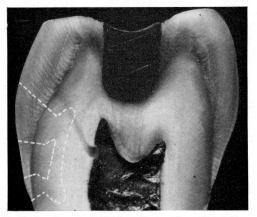

Fig. 45. Occlusal and gingival walls in Class V cavity are cut parallel to the general direction of the enamel prisms.

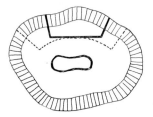

Fig. 46. Mesial and distal walls of Class V cavity are cut parallel to the general direction of the enamel prisms.

The retention grooves are cut in the dentine of the axio-gingival and axio-occlusal line angles, sufficiently away from the amelo-dentinal junction not to leave unsupported enamel (*Fig.* 45). No attempt is made to undercut the dentine mesially and distally, as this will tend to weaken the tooth tissue at the angles of the cavity (*Fig.* 46).

In Class V cavities which are narrow occluso-gingivally, adequate retention can be obtained with an inverted cone burr (*Fig.* 47). However, if the occluso-gingival width has had to be greatly

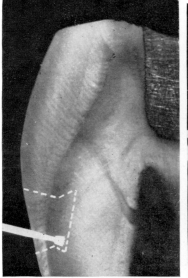 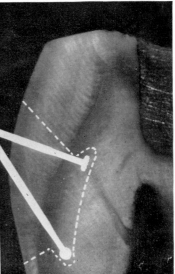

Fig. 47. Inverted cone burr providing retention in occlusal and gingival walls of Class V cavity.

Fig. 48. Retention grooves cut in occlusal and gingival walls of extensive Class V cavity with wheel burr and round burr respectively.

increased, then the occlusal and gingival walls will form a more obtuse angle in order to avoid the leaving of weak unsupported enamel. The resulting wide cavity, with markedly divergent walls, will in all probability not be adequately restored with amalgam retained by the small occlusal and gingival undercuts formed by an inverted cone burr.

Markley (1955) recommends using a large wheel burr in enlarging the axio-occlusal retention groove, and a No. 1 round burr for the axio-gingival retention groove (*Fig.* 48). These burrs will facilitate adequate access to the cavity and allow for cutting the retention grooves at the level of the axial wall, and so avoid any risk of undermining the enamel. Markley stresses that it is important to ensure that the amalgam is properly condensed into these retention grooves with narrow bladed pluggers, otherwise the grooves serve merely as mercury traps. Care should be taken when lining these cavities not to reduce or obliterate these retention grooves.

There is some divergence of opinion over the shape of the axial wall. Markley (1955) recommends that the axial wall should be as flat as possible in a mesiodistal direction (*Fig.* 49). This, of course, would result in the cavity being deeper at the centre than at the mesial and distal ends. He suggests a flat axial floor in order to reduce the likelihood of the amalgam, during condensation, sliding out of the cavity as successive layers are condensed.

Pickard (1973), however, recommends that the depth of the axial floor should be uniform, so resulting in a convex axial wall (*Fig.* 49). This approach has the advantage of being more conservative of

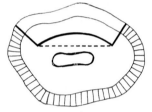

Fig. 49. Comparison of curved and flat axial walls to Class V cavity.

tooth tissue and therefore less injurious to the pulp. The amalgam can be prevented from sliding out of the cavity during condensation, by using a matrix band having a window cut in it large enough for adequate insertion and condensation of the amalgam. The latter more conservative approach is to be preferred.

The axial wall in an occluso-gingival direction is usually kept flat (*Fig.* 47), except where the width is excessive, and then a slightly convex axial wall is preferred (*Fig.* 48).

Auxiliary Retention

It is not always possible to obtain adequate retention for amalgam restorations by either occlusally convergent walls or by undercutting the remaining tooth tissue. Either there is inadequate tooth tissue to support the amalgam restoration, or adequate provision for retention would result in excessive weakening of the remaining tooth structure. In either case the resistance form of the restored tooth would be poor.

Auxiliary retention of amalgam restorations must not be confused with attempts to improve the resistance form of either the amalgam restoration or residual tooth tissue. The object is to aid retention of the restoration without reducing the resistance form of the remaining tooth tissue or the restoration. In an attempt to improve the strength of the amalgam restoration where cavity design would have resulted in poor resistance form, Bull (1936) advocated using 90 per cent silver plate cut roughly to the size and shape of the cavity to reinforce amalgam restorations. Here the technique consisted of condensing amalgam as an initial layer into the cavity, and then tapping the shaped piece of silver plate home in the amalgam. Then successive layers of amalgam are condensed over the plate. In very large cavities several alternating layers of amalgam and silver plate could be inserted. Petersen and Freedman (1972) experimented with reinforcing silver amalgam using ductile metal laminates in regions of the restoration that are subjected to tensile forces. They showed that by incorporating silver plated stainless-steel laminates of 0·0015 in thickness into an amalgam restoration the transverse strength was increased considerably. The silver plating of the stainless steel facilitates bonding with the amalgam matrix which does not attack the stainless steel. However, since surface cracks appear in the amalgam at lower transverse strength measurements, although these do not go through the laminate, it is questionable whether there is a clinical value in such reinforcing techniques.

Auxiliary retention of amalgam restorations can be achieved by using cemented pins, friction-retained pins or self-tapping pins. With all pin techniques isolation of the tooth with rubber dam will eliminate the risk of the patient inhaling or swallowing a pin.

Cement-retained Pins
The earliest techniques of achieving amalgam retention with cemented pins involved using stainless-steel orthodontic wire matched to slightly larger diameter round or flat fissure burrs (*Fig. 50*); the essential points of the technique being that the hole is drilled in the dentine just within the amelo-dentinal junction (*Fig. 51*) to a depth of 2–3 mm and a small length of contoured ortho-dontic wire is cemented into place. Some practitioners sandblast the orthodontic wire in order to roughen the surface. A further development was the introduction of the D.M. Co. Platinoid threaded German silver wire (*Fig. 52*) which is produced in $1\frac{1}{2}$ in lengths. Here one was able either to cement short lengths of wire into holes prepared with a No. $\frac{1}{2}$ fissure burr, or screw and subse-quently cut off the wire in smaller diameter holes. Pickard (1973) suggests screwing these dentine pins home in holes drilled by a

31

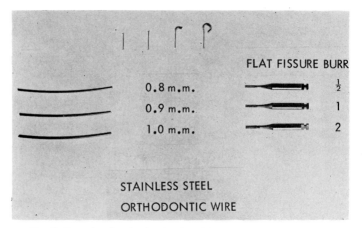

FLAT FISSURE BURR

0.8 m.m.   ½

0.9 m.m.   1

1.0 m.m.   2

STAINLESS STEEL

ORTHODONTIC WIRE

Fig. 50. Lengths of orthodontic wire with matched flat fissure burrs, with sections cut and contoured prior to cementation.

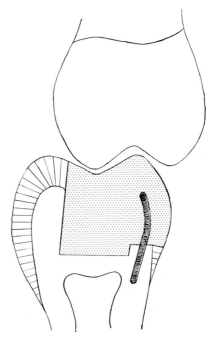

Fig. 51. Auxiliary retention of amalgam provided by a dentine pin. *Note* (*a*) pin in dentine is parallel to outer contour of tooth; (*b*) pin in amalgam follows contour of cusp of amalgam restoration.

32

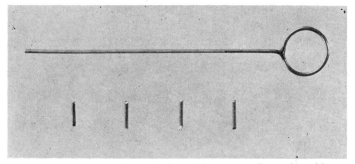

Fig. 52. D.M. Co. Platinoid threaded German silver wire with sections cut prior to cementation.

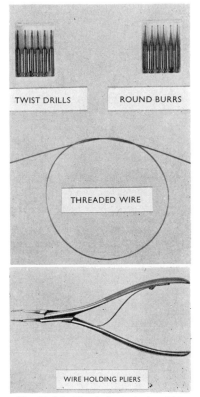

Fig. 53. Markley 'wire technique' kit.

$\frac{1}{4}$ round burr but this can prove a very difficult procedure especially with the full length of wire in posterior teeth.

Markley (1958) has very ably illustrated how successfully teeth

33

which otherwise would be unsavable can be restored with amalgam by using cemented lengths of threaded wrought metal wire and the method he described is now the most standardized of the cemented pin techniques (*Fig.* 53). The advantage of the dentine pin is that its thinness allows room for several pins, if necessary, to be inserted into a cavity, the number used being dependent on the amount of tooth tissue lost; if the path of insertion of each pin is varied one to another, the retention of the filling will be enhanced once the amalgam which is packed around them has hardened (*Fig.* 54). An attempt to improve amalgam retention by excessively changing the path of insertion of the pins one to another can lead to perforation of the pulp or periodontal ligament.

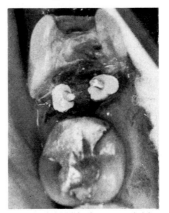

Fig. 54. Dentine pins cemented in large mesial box. Note different angles at which pins project into cavity.

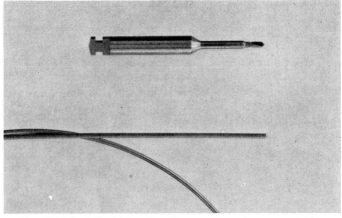

Fig. 55. Twist drill with 'stop' at $2\frac{1}{2}$ mm to prevent over-penetration of burr.

The essential components of the Markley pin system are the matched twist drill and wire (*Fig. 55*). The twist drill comes in diameters of 0·021 in for anterior teeth and 0·027 in for posterior teeth with the wire 0·019 in and 0·025 in respectively to allow for cementation.

The stages of the technique are:

1. Make a small depression or starting point in the dentine adjacent to the amelo-dentinal junction using a ½ round burr. This will prevent the twist drill slipping on the dentine face.

2. Using an 0·021 in or 0·027 in twist drill depending on the diameter of the wire to be cemented, drill a hole to a depth of 2½ mm in the dentine parallel to the adjacent outer contour of the tooth. A knowledge of tooth morphology aided by X-rays will prevent perforating the pulp or periodontal ligament. In the case of Class V cavities, the pins are inserted at the mesial and distal ends of the cavity to avoid the pulp (*Fig. 56*).

3. The end of the threaded wire should be rounded with a sandpaper disc in order to facilitate the wire being pushed to the full depth of the pin hole, and the wire is then cut with wire cutters to desired length.

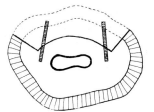

Fig. 56. Auxiliary retention in large Class V cavities provided by dentine pins placed mesially and distally at variant angles.

4. Insert the smooth end of the cut length of wire into the pin hole and check that the length does not interfere with the occlusion.

5. Remove the wire and bend with pliers to follow the approximate outer contour of the amalgam restoration (*see Fig. 51*).

6. After ensuring that the pin hole is clean and dry, either insert a creamy mix of zinc phosphate cement into the pin hole with a straight probe or lentulo spiral, or liberally 'butter' the rounded end of the pin and insert the pin to the full depth of the pin hole. This latter method is easier in the multi-pinned restoration, otherwise there is the additional problem of finding the pin holes with the excess cement around the openings, and also the risk of the cement beginning to set before all the pins are seated. It is important also to ensure that the contoured pins are rotated to their correct position.

35

7. When the cement has set the excess cement can be easily removed with a sharp probe or excavator.

Friction-retained Pins
Essentially this technique consists of drilling a hole into the dentine which is slightly smaller in diameter than the pin to be inserted.

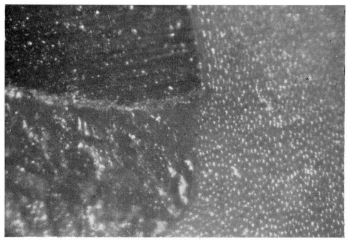

Fig. 57. Photomicrograph of section of friction-retained pin in dentine. Note compression of dentinal tubules adjacent to pin and presence of step below end of pin. Space below pin and base of pin hole filled with debris. (*By courtesy of J. M. Richards.*)

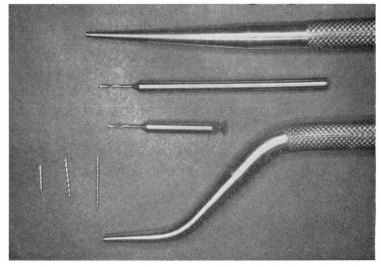

Fig. 58. Unitek system for friction-retained pins.

The pin is gently pushed or tapped home in the pin hole, the elasticity of the dentine allowing the slightly over-sized pin to seat and then maintain a frictional grip of the pin (*Fig. 57*).

Goldstein (1966) reported the use of the friction-locked pin kit manufactured by Unitek Corporation of California (*Fig. 58*) and subsequently Weil of Toronto manufactured an alternative friction retained pin kit (*Fig. 59*). These kits consist of 0·021 in twist drills and pre-cut lengths of 0·022 in stainless-steel wire.

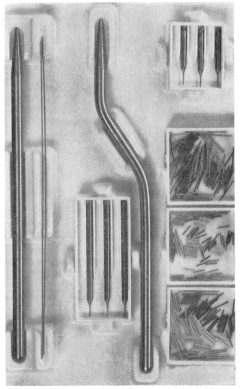

Fig. 59. Weil system for friction-retained pins.

The stages of the technique are:

1. Make a starting point in dentine with a $\frac{1}{2}$ round burr approximately 1 mm from the amelo-dentinal junction. It is important to ensure that there is an adequate bulk of dentine between the pin hole and the amelo-dentinal junction. A pin hole drilled too close to the amelo-dentinal junction may lead to fracture of the cavity margin adjacent to the pin hole, as a result of the stress produced when forcing the pin home.

37

2. Using a 0·021 in twist drill, prepare a pin hole to the depth of 2–3 mm in the dentine, parallel to the adjacent outer contour of the tooth.

3. Select a suitable pre-cut length of pin and insert this in the pin setter. The bayonet or offset pin setter should be used for posterior teeth (*Fig*. 58). A calibrated periodontal probe will aid the choice of length of precut pin which the manufacturers produce in three lengths.

4. Ensure that the pin hole is clean and dry and with the aid of the pin setter insert the pin into the pin hole. Hand force is usually adequate but gently tapping the pin setter will aid seating the pin.

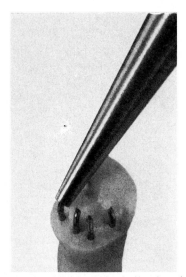

Fig. 60. Bending friction-retained pin using pin setter.

5. Using the pin setter, bend the pin towards the centre of the cavity to increase the thickness of the amalgam around the pin and allow access for amalgam pluggers between the pin and matrix band. The pin setter should be raised about 1 mm from the dentine surface when bending the pin in order to reduce lateral stress on the dentine. The lip of the pin setter acts as a fulcrum for bending the pin rather than the point of entry of the pin in the dentine (*Fig*. 60).

6. Check the occlusion and, if necessary, excess length of pin can be removed with a water-cooled high-speed round diamond burr working from the end of the pin. No attempt should be made to section off the excess length as the pin can be loosened and become a dangerous projectile. Removal of the pin with pliers, sectioning excess length outside the mouth and reinserting the pin in the same

pin hole, often results in reduced retention of the pin. If the pin is removed it is better to drill a new hole for its reinsertion.

Screw-retained Pins

Going (1966) has described the technique of using self-tapping gold-plated stainless-steel screws for aiding the retention of silver amalgam. This is known as the Threadmate system (T.M.S.) manufactured by Whaledent Inc. Essentially the technique consists of using a threaded pin (*Fig.* 61) slightly larger than the pin hole and

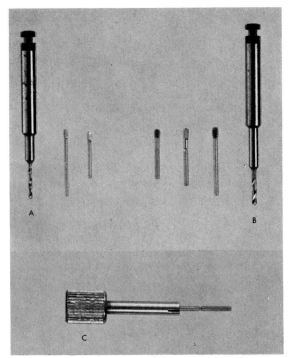

Fig. 61. T.M.S. screw-retained pin system. A, 0·021 in twist drill and matched screws; B, 0·027 in twist drill and matched screws; C, Hand wrench for screwing pin into dentine.

seating it by screwing it home; the pin produces its own thread in the dentine. The pins are screwed home by means of a hand wrench which fits over the flattened end of the screw. Alternatively, the pin can be placed in the pin hole by a special chuck that fits into a reduction gear handpiece (*Fig.* 62). Previously, Dentatus screws (*Fig.* 63) had been used but because of their size it was difficult to insert them para-pulpally without the risk of damage to the pulp or the periodontal ligament. In root-filled teeth Dentatus screws can be inserted into the root canal and so aid retention of the amalgam restoration (Nicholls, 1963).

The stages of the technique are:

1. Make a starting point in the dentine with a $\frac{1}{2}$ round burr approximately 1 mm from the amelo-dentinal junction. Again avoid being too close to the amelo-dentinal junction.

2. Using a 0·021 in or 0·027 in twist drill, depending on the diameter of the screw to be used, drill a hole to a depth of 2–3 mm in the dentine parallel to the adjacent outer contour of the tooth.

3. Ensure that the pin hole is clean and dry and, after inserting the pin in the hand wrench, screw the pin to the full depth of the pin hole.

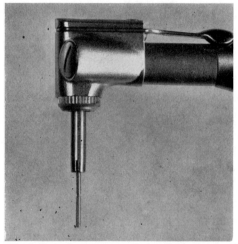

Fig. 62. 10 : 1 Reducing contra-angle handpiece head with chuck holding two-in-one T.M.S. pin.

A 10 : 1 reducing gear auto-clutch handpiece with a special chuck can be used for screwing the pin home. Three types of pin are available for each diameter size: 7 mm length pin where the flattened head remains attached to the threaded part of the pin; 8 mm two-in-one pin which breaks into two 4 mm lengths after the first half has been screwed home; 5 mm self-shearing pin where the flattened head breaks away from the threaded part of the pin when the pin is fully seated, due to the increased strain of screwing which results in fracture at the weakened junction of head and pin.

4. Check the occlusion and if necessary remove excess length of pin 'fouling the bite' with a water-cooled high-speed air-rotor round diamond burr. If the flattened head of the pin is still attached to the threaded part, the pin can be unscrewed, excess length removed with wire cutters and the pin replaced after rounding the sectioned end with a sandpaper disc.

5. Contour the pin with the bending tool (*Fig.* 64) to follow the approximate contour of the restoration so that there is an adequate bulk of amalgam around the pin. As in the case of the friction-

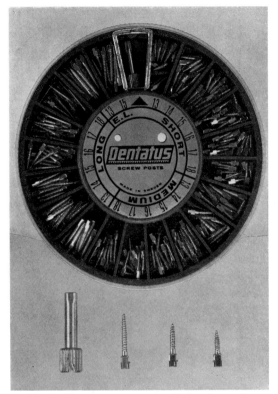

Fig. 63. Dentatus screw posts with hand wrench.

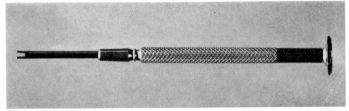

Fig. 64. Bending tool for T.M.S. pin.

retained pin, care must be exercised to prevent fracturing the cavity margin when bending the located pin. By using the two-pronged bending tool, a fulcrum is provided by one of the prongs over which

41

the wire is bent by the other prong (*Fig.* 65). Care must be taken to ensure that the pin has not been bent into a position where it interferes with the occlusion.

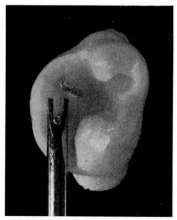

Fig. 65. Bending T.M.S. pin, centrally placed prong acting as fulcrum.

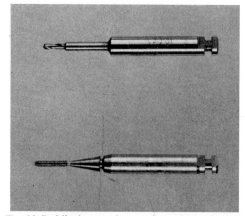

Fig. 66. Stabilock screw burr and matched twist drill.

More recently a simplified screw-retained system has been marketed where the self-tapping screw is the terminal part of a burr fitting into the standard contra-angle handpiece (*Fig.* 66). After preparing the pin hole with the provided matched twist drill, the screw burr is drilled into the pin hole. The terminal screw breaks away from the burr when the torque force is greater than the weakened junction of screw and burr. It has yet to be established if the

42

screw is in fact at the full depth of the pin hole before the junction of the screw and burr fractures. In addition, the screw cannot be contoured.

Dilts et al. (1968) experimented on the forces needed to remove pins inserted into dentine at various depths and using different pin techniques. They showed that: (a) the greatest retention in dentine is with self-threading pins, (b) in the case of the cement-retained pin, zinc phosphate provides the greatest retention of the three cementing media investigated, namely, calcium hydroxide, zinc oxide/eugenol and zinc phosphate, (c) the optimum depth of the pin in dentine is from 2–3 mm for self-tapping pins and 3–4 mm for cemented pins. The main advantages of the cemented pin system is that there is no stress on the dentine during insertion or contouring of the pin and in addition the pin can be altered in length and contour before cementation. The practitioner must decide whether these advantages outweigh its relatively poorer retention in dentine, the risk of pulpal irritation from the zinc phosphate cement, and the risk of easier dislodgement during amalgam condensation procedures.

Wing (1965) and Duperon and Kasloff (1971) have evaluated the relative compressive strength of amalgam to the number of pins inserted. They have shown that regardless of the type of pin systems used, as the number of pins inserted into the amalgam increased so the compressive strength of the amalgam diminished. It is thought that stress concentrations in the amalgam are built up at the serrations as well as at the wire itself (*Fig.* 67) which result in the weakening of the amalgam. This is supported by studies with photo-elastic stress analyses.

In addition, Welk and Dilts (1967) investigated not only the retentive strength of the various pin systems in dentine but also that in amalgam. They have suggested that there is little value in having the relative retentive strength of the pin in amalgam greater than its retentive strength in dentine. Having established that the pins weaken amalgam, they have shown that for an optimum penetration of 3 mm of the cemented pin in dentine the pin should penetrate 1 mm into amalgam to give equivalent retentive strength. A penetration of 2 mm into amalgam provided greater retentive strength in the amalgam. When the threaded pin is screw-retained in dentine, then for an optimum retentive strength value of 2 mm penetration into dentine, the pin should penetrate 2 mm into amalgam to give equivalent retention. Friction-retained pins provided the least retentive strength values in amalgam of all the pin systems and would require a penetration in amalgam of over 6 mm to approach the retentive strength values of the threaded pins.

From the foregoing it must be clear that pins do not reinforce the amalgam restoration but only provide retention. It behoves the

43

practitioner to use the minimum number of pins with optimum depth in dentine and amalgam to provide the retention necessary to restore the tooth.

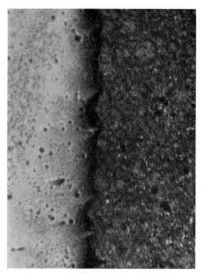

Fig. 67. Photomicrograph of serrated wire in amalgam. Stress concentrations build up at these serrations.

3. REMOVAL OF PULPAL CARIES

In small cavities it is commonly unnecessary to make this a separate step in cavity preparation, as the previous stages of establishing the outline form and the resistance and retention forms will have removed all the remaining carious dentine.

Gabel (1954) recommends the removal of caries before establishing the resistance and retention form of the cavity, in order to get any necessary obtundent solutions to the dentine, as they will not pass through the caries. Also, any carious involvement of the pulp can be established at an early stage.

However, Black (1947), McGehee et al. (1956), Pickard (1973), and many others advocate no cutting toward the pulp until the cavity is practically completed, so that if there is pulpal involvement the necessary pulp treatment can be instituted without risking additional contamination of the pulp from further cavity preparation.

The pulpal caries should be removed with sharp excavators by loosening around the margins of the caries and peeling it up, so that pressure is directed away from the pulp. Burrs should not be used.

44

It should be noted that it is good practice to leave hard, stained dentine in the pulpal floor or axial wall of a cavity, which in the clinical judgement of the operator is in close proximity to the pulp. This is provided that no more caries can be removed with sharp excavators, and that the previous history of the tooth does not suggest irreparable pulpal involvement. There is, however, considerable discussion as to whether it is permissible to leave soft caries in the pulpal floor of a cavity.

Romnes (1953) and many others are quite categoric about removing all caries, and consider the leaving of caries questionable practice. However, De Boer (1956), whilst stressing the fact that all caries in the amelo-dentinal junction area must be removed down to hard dentine, reminds us of the work done by Kraus (1945, 1952), Batt (1942), and Besic (1943), who have supported the principle of leaving caries over the pulp, a method known as 'indirect pulp capping'.

Shovelton (1972), in reviewing the histological and bacteriological studies of the deep carious lesion, has clearly shown the efficacy of indirect pulp capping in maintaining pulp vitality. The technique requires that the cavity preparation procedures of establishing correct outline, resistance and retention forms are followed but the total removal of caries with the attendant risk of pulpal exposure is avoided. The subsequent treatment of the cavity before restoring with amalgam is discussed later under 'Lining in very deep cavities' (*see Fig.* 74).

4. CONVENIENCE FORM

'Convenience form' is the term applied in cavity preparation to the shape given to a cavity to provide reasonable access for the removal of caries and allow instrumentation required for lining and filling the cavity.

Having established the general form of the cavity, it is sometimes necessary to modify the cavity in order to facilitate:

a. A clear sight of the deeper aspects of the cavity;

b. An easier approach to all the internal surfaces and angles of the cavity with burrs and chisels;

c. A proper condensation of the restorative material.

Modification of the cavity to establish convenience form is rarely necessary in teeth to be restored with amalgam, since the correct preparation of outline and resistance and retention forms will automatically result in proper convenience form.

In fact, the need for convenience form as a separate step in cavity preparation originates in those procedures which facilitate the condensing of cohesive gold foil.

5. FINISHING OF THE ENAMEL WALLS AND MARGINS

The two main factors which control the finishing of the enamel wall are:

a. The direction of the enamel rods;

b. The edge strength of the restorative material.

The enamel wall of the cavity must be cut so that all enamel rods are supported by sound dentine. It is for this reason that the mesial and distal walls of a Class V cavity are divergent from the floor of the cavity (*see Fig.* 46), while the walls of a Class I cavity, especially under the cusps, can be occlusally convergent (*see Fig.* 37). Thus it will be seen that the inclination of the enamel wall is to a certain extent controlled by the location of the cavity in the tooth.

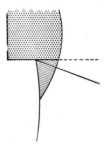

Fig. 68. Area between extended lines shows area of unsupported enamel at cavo-gingival line angle.

It should be stressed that the weak edge strength of amalgam prevents the use of the short bevel at the cavo-surface line angle. The inadvertent short bevel is probably the most common cause of the 'ditched' amalgam restoration (*see Fig.* 2). This short bevel is very easily produced if the burr is not cutting along its whole length, or if sandpaper discs are used to finish the enamel walls of amalgam cavities. Ideally, the enamel wall should be finished with sharp chisels in a planing action along the whole depth of the walls of the cavity, so as to remove any broken or unsupported enamel prisms.

With regard to the finishing of the cavo-gingival line angle, it can be seen in *Fig.* 68 that, as the gingival floor is cut at right angles to the vertical occlusal stress, an extension of this horizontal plane to the cavo-gingival line angle would result in leaving unsupported enamel.

This unsupported enamel must be removed, otherwise subsequent fracture of the prisms will result in a nidus for recurrent caries. The removal of the gingival unsupported enamel is often referred to as 'bevelling the cavo-gingival line angle'. This term is strictly incorrect,

46

since the result of removing the unsupported enamel rods is to produce an enamel wall parallel to the direction of the prisms, and not to cut and so protect the superficial ends of the dentine-supported enamel rods. Markley (1951) has suggested producing a 20° bevel of the gingival enamel wall, but Link (1944) and Romnes (1953) prefer the more commonly accepted procedure of planing the gingival enamel wall with Black's gingival margin trimmers (*Fig.* 69). This will, in addition to removing undermined enamel prisms, also produce a butt joint between the amalgam and enamel walls.

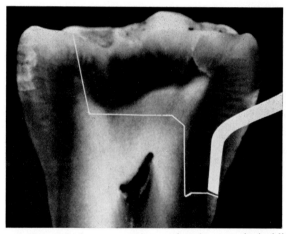

Fig. 69. Removal of unsupported enamel at the cavo-gingival line angle using a Black gingival margin trimmer.

However, Boyde et al. (1972) have shown with their scanning electron microscope studies that, in fact, the use of chisels normally available to dental practitioners to finish enamel walls in cavity preparations results in the smearing of enamel tissue (*Fig.* 70). This is due to the enamel being removed from one area, distorted and welded to another area as a result of the local high pressure and temperature. In a more recent study Boyde (1973) has shown that by using specially prepared tungsten-carbide tipped chisels it was possible to produce a neat cavity margin with reduced smearing (*Fig.* 71).

Baker and Curson (1974) have demonstrated that a high standard of cavity margin finish can be achieved by using a modified tungsten-carbide burr run at ultra-high speed in the air turbine handpiece. The modified burr is produced by grinding away the terminal blades of a standard tungsten-carbide end-cutting burr and subsequently contouring the resultant blank on a diamond burr. They have shown

47

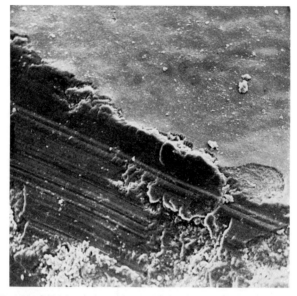

Fig. 70. S.E.M. section of enamel finished with chisel showing smeared surface. (*By courtesy of Dr A. Boyde.*)

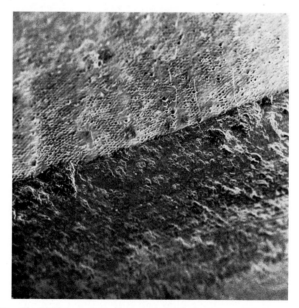

Fig. 71. S.E.M. section of enamel finished with special tungsten-carbide chisel. (*By courtesy of Dr A.Boyde.*)

by scanning electron microscopy studies that the abrasive action of the very fine tungsten-carbide particles, left on the surface of the modified burr, produces a finish to the enamel surface comparable to the best obtainable.

6. CAVITY TOILET

The purpose of this step is to remove all debris and loose particles that may remain in the cavity as a result of the procedures of cavity preparation, leaving the cavity absolutely clean. This will allow the lining and amalgam to be placed against clean cavity walls.

Another aspect of cavity toilet is the questionable need of sterilizing the cavity. Zander (1940) has shown the presence of organisms remaining in well-prepared cavities. Fisher (1969) reviewed the fate of organisms left in the dentine under fillings and showed that organisms such as lactobacilli and anaerobic streptococci could remain viable under non-antiseptic fillings for long periods of time. However, in a more recent study Fisher (1972) has demonstrated that viable micro-organisms are not recoverable from previously infected dentine which has been covered by calcium hydroxide as a sub-base under a lining of zinc phosphate and amalgam. Jordan and Suzuki (1971) have produced similar results with zinc oxide/eugenol type liners.

Although there is some question as to whether drugs will produce sterility of dentine at the time of cavity preparation, there is little doubt that some of the drugs commonly used in cavity toilet will produce harmful effects on the pulp. Zander (1954) has stated that the two main drawbacks of drugs for cavity sterilization are: (a) pulpal irritation; (b) alteration of the permeability of the dentine. The degree of irritation depends on whether escharotic drugs such as silver nitrate, phenol, etc., are used, or more mild solutions such as eugenol or thymol, and also on the proximity of the floor of the cavity to the pulp.

Work done by Amler (1948) has shown that the treatment of dentine with drugs such as phenol, silver nitrate or alcohol results in an increased permeability of the dentine, and that in any event these drugs do not form the barrier between pulp and filling material that has been claimed.

Although the use of obtundent drugs may affect the sensitivity of the dentine by coagulating the superficial contents of the dentinal tubules, Zander (1954) claims that it is the resultant shrinkage of the protoplasmic processes which allows for the increased permeability of the dentine.

Cavity sterilization at the time of cavity preparation is contra-indicated, therefore, for the following reasons:

a. It is not possible to sterilize the dentine completely at the time of cavity preparation without damage to a vital pulp;

b. It is doubtful if the isolated organisms which may remain in a properly prepared and restored cavity can be harmful;

c. The lining materials, such as calcium hydroxide in very deep cavities and zinc oxide/eugenol in deep cavities, have been shown to produce sterilization of the dentine over a period of time.

It can be seen from the foregoing that the cavity should not be swabbed with drugs, but debris lying in the internal angles of the cavity should be dislodged with a probe and washed out of the cavity with atomized warm water. The cavity is then dried with warm air and pledgets of cotton-wool before lining, care being taken not to dehydrate the dentine.

CHAPTER 3

LINING OF AMALGAM RESTORATIONS

IT must first be noted that, although the pulp has an ability to resist injury and to repair itself, this is limited, and it is the responsibility of the dentist to keep any untoward stimulation of the pulp to a minimum. This is done by careful cavity preparation and adequate protection of the pulp from harmful stimuli from or through the restoration.

In teeth to be restored with amalgam, pulpal trauma can commonly result from:

1. Initial bacterial invasion from the carious lesions.

2. Cutting trauma during cavity preparation—as in deep cavities resulting in near or actual exposures.

3. Thermal trauma resulting from:

   a. Heat generated by cavity preparation;

   b. Heat generated by excessive polishing of the amalgam restoration;

   c. Temperature changes conducted through the restoration from excessively hot or cold foods or fluids.

4. Chemical trauma resulting from:

   a. Some cavity sterilization drugs, e.g. phenol, silver nitrate;

   b. Some lining materials, e.g. zinc phosphate cement.

5. Electrical trauma resulting from galvanic current generated by opposing dissimilar restorations coming into contact at the make and break of that contact.

Thanik et al. (1962) have shown that minute pulp exposures cannot be clinically detected, and therefore in all deep cavities one must suspect the existence of near or frank exposures. It is for this reason that it is essential in very deep cavities to protect the pulp with a non-irritating base material. They have shown in a comparison of the relative toxicities of zinc phosphate, zinc oxide/eugenol, and calcium hydroxide bases that zinc phosphate is, in fact, very irritating, zinc oxide/eugenol mildly irritating, and calcium hydroxide non-irritating to the pulp. In point of fact, calcium hydroxide, which has a high alkalinity, is not a completely bland material. Berman (1958) has suggested that calcium hydroxide produces the primary calcific bridge over the exposed pulp by producing a rapid necrosis and degeneration of the superficial layers of the pulp.

51

Lyell (1960) explains why zinc phosphate, notwithstanding its known harmful effect on the pulp, is still used as a lining material. This is due to the relatively higher compressive strength of zinc phosphate cement, which will allow adequate packing pressures for amalgam condensation without itself fracturing under the load. However, Plant and Wilson (1971) have demonstrated that during condensation of conventional alloys, the maximum stress transmitted to a lining is 26 N/mm^2 (3,770 lb/sq in) and for spherical alloys 17 N/mm^2 (2,465 lb/sq in). These results, considered with their previous work (Plant and Wilson, 1970) on the early strength of lining materials, show that quick-setting zinc oxide/eugenol type liners as well as zinc polycarboxylate and zinc phosphate cements, will be strong enough to withstand these condensing forces provided they have set. The condensation technique followed will greatly affect the compressive strength required of a lining material; for example, the Eames minimal mercury technique, requiring a hand condensation thrust of 3–6 lb (13–27 N), will be less traumatic on a lining than a hand condensation thrust of 8–10 lb (36–45 N). Phillips (1963) suggests that the subsequent fracture of amalgam restorations is more commonly due to incorrect occlusal relationships rather than an insufficient strength of the underlying base, and supports the concept that the purpose of a lining material is primarily one of insulation against thermal and chemical insult. In addition, a lining can serve the purpose of reducing an oversize cavity to a more classical shape and depth (*see Fig.* 6). This will avoid the risk of cuspal fracture resulting from thermal expansion of an excessive bulk of amalgam.

In an attempt to make zinc phosphate cements stronger, some practitioners have mixed particles of amalgam alloy with the zinc phosphate cement. Mahler and Armen (1962) have investigated the improvement in the properties of zinc phosphate cement having alloy particles added. They have found that, although there is no improvement in compressive strength, there is an improvement in the transverse or sheer strength of the zinc phosphate cement; the more the particles of amalgam alloy and the larger their size, the greater the increase in transverse strength. There is, however, no better adhesion to dentine, although there is a greater resistance to dissolution.

The clinical advantage of this amalgam alloy/zinc phosphate cement mixture is as a temporary filling or for blanking out undercuts in extra-coronal gold restorations. It is doubtful whether it increases the efficiency of amalgam restorations, to have such a lining. This must not be confused with the 'Baldwin technique' used by some practitioners in the fond hope of obtaining better retention for the amalgam restoration. This technique, originally described by

Baldwin (1897), consists of condensing amalgam on to unset zinc phosphate cement so that the cement adheres to the amalgam and cavity walls.

With regard to thermal insulation, work done by Braden (1964) has shown that the problem of insulating the pulp from thermal stimuli conveyed via the metal filling is one of transient heat conduction, as distinct from a steady state. He has shown that the physical property concerned in evaluating the efficiency of thermal insulation is the thermal diffusivity of the lining material rather than its thermal conductivity.

Braden has shown that there are only minor differences between the respective thermal diffusivities of dentine, zinc phosphate cement and zinc oxide/eugenol cement. Furthermore, in the case of zinc phosphate and zinc oxide/eugenol cements their values are relatively insensitive to variations in their liquid/powder ratios. However, since the rate of temperature change through a lining increases in proportion to the lining thickness squared, it follows that variations in lining thickness have much more influence on the efficacy of thermal insulation than the physical properties of either of these lining materials.

The knowledge that dentine has relatively the same thermal insulating power as zinc phosphate or zinc oxide/eugenol cements supports the currently held practice of not deepening a cavity which is just through the amelo-dentinal junction to make room for a lining under an amalgam restoration. However, there still remains the problem of dentine sensitivity and the need for sealing the dentinal tubules.

Much research has been done in the last ten years on the ability of amalgam to seal the cavity from the ingress of saliva. The consensus of opinion of workers is that marginal leakage does take place around an amalgam restoration, but that this marginal percolation is most marked initially and decreases as the restoration ages. This, it has been argued, is due to the dissociated metallic ions and corrosive products slowly filling the space (Nelsen et al., 1952; Going et al., 1960; Swartz and Phillips, 1961, 1962).

Going and Massler (1961) have shown that zinc phosphate provides a poor seal under silver amalgam restorations, and, in fact, increased the marginal penetration of the isotope used in their experiments; this, they argue, is caused by the effect of the phosphoric acid of the zinc phosphate cement on the dentine. They have also shown an increased permeability between the cement and amalgam, which they claim is due to the acid etching the amalgam surface with which it is in contact. Phillips et al. (1955) have shown that zinc phosphate is, in addition, not as efficient an insulator against galvanic stimuli when compared with zinc oxide/eugenol base.

53

Von Fraunhofer and Staheli (1972) report that galvanic current generated through contact between gold and amalgam in the mouth is of sufficient magnitude to run a deaf aid or small transmitter and could well contribute to pulpal irritation.

The foregoing evidence must therefore bring into question the wisdom of using zinc phosphate as an intermediary base between amalgam and dentine. Smith (1968) has been responsible for developing a new dental cement based on a modified zinc oxide and an aqueous solution of polyacrylic acid to produce a zinc polycarboxylate matrix, made up by the cross-linking of adjacent polyacrylic acid molecules by zinc ions. The main clinical advantage of this material is its relatively greater adhesion to dentine and enamel than any other dental cement. It has been shown to have a lower compressive but greater tensile strength than zinc phosphate cement. However, Plant (1970) has demonstrated its irritant effect on the pulp which must question its use as a sole base between amalgam and dentine. Quick-setting zinc oxide/eugenol, on the other hand, has been shown by Swartz and Phillips (1962) to provide a good seal against marginal leakage and to act as a good thermal and electrical insulator. In addition, the eugenol has mildly antiseptic and obtundent properties, so having a therapeutic effect on the freshly cut dentinal tubules. The addition of ethoxybenzoic acid (E.B.A.), polymers and alumina have increased the strength of zinc oxide/eugenol cements. However, these reinforced zinc oxide/eugenol cements are not as strong as zinc phosphate cement.

There is also much in the literature on cavity varnishes and liners. The varnishes consist principally of either a synthetic or natural resin (for example, rosin or copal respectively) dissolved in a volatile solvent such as chloroform, acetone or ether. The liners usually consist of suspensions of calcium hydroxide, either in distilled water or in organic solvent solutions such as methyl cellulose. While the varnishes have been shown by Swartz and Phillips (1962) to eliminate marginal percolation around amalgam restorations, their inefficiency as thermal and electrical insulators in deep cavities would require their use to be in conjunction with an intermediate base.

It has been previously pointed out that calcium hydroxide is the least irritating of cement bases, and that it facilitates the formation of a secondary dentine bridge over an exposed pulp (Berman, 1958; Thanik et al., 1962). However, Phillips et al. (1955) have shown calcium hydroxide to be ineffective as a galvanic current insulator, and it certainly does not become sufficiently hard or strong to be a sole base under an amalgam restoration. Since it does act as an efficient barrier against phosphoric acid, it can be covered with zinc phosphate cement to provide a lining of adequate thickness.

For the purposes of the type of lining to be used, cavities can be divided into three types:

1. *Shallow Cavities*
Where the cavity is cut to about 1 mm into dentine. This is an ideal depth, where there will be minimal pulpal trauma, while at the same time allowing for adequate resistance and retention form. No lining is required other than a cavity varnish (*Fig.* 72). This will provide an adequate protective seal which has been shown to be necessary by Granath and Möller (1971) who investigated the biological effect on human dental pulp of silver amalgam in shallow cavities and demonstrated a high incidence of mild pulpal inflammation when there is no lining.

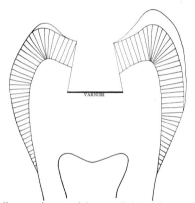

Fig. 72. Shallow cavity requiring no lining other than a varnish.

The varnish should cover the enamel wall as well as the dentine since it has been shown to reduce marginal leakage around freshly inserted amalgam. Subsequent loss of this peripheral varnish appears to be compensated for by the corrosive products of the amalgam sealing the amalgam enamel interface.

2. *Deep Cavities*
Where caries requires the cavity to be deepened farther, a lining of quick-setting zinc oxide/eugenol is preferred (*Fig.* 73). Hoppenstand and McConnell (1960) have shown that a zinc oxide/eugenol base is as strong as a zinc phosphate base, provided that the amalgam restoration is partly supported in sound dentine. That is to say, that only those parts of the cavity which have had to be deepened for caries removal are lined with the quick-setting zinc oxide/eugenol base, and the rest of the cavity floor, which has been cut to about 1 mm into dentine, is left unlined, other than being covered by a layer of varnish.

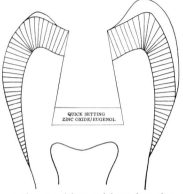

Fig. 73. Deep cavity requiring quick-setting zinc oxide/eugenol type lining.

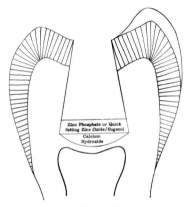

Fig. 74. Very deep cavity requiring pulpal protection with sub-base of calcium hydroxide and lining of quick-setting zinc oxide/eugenol type cement or zinc phosphate cement.

3. *Very Deep Cavities*

Since one must consider the likelihood of microscopic exposures in very deep cavities, these cavities must always first be lined with a layer of calcium hydroxide (*Fig.* 74). The calcium hydroxide can then be covered with a second lining of zinc phosphate, zinc poly-carboxylate or quick-setting zinc oxide/eugenol cement. A thin coating of varnish is then applied by placing a small amount in the cavity and spreading it as a thin film by means of an air blast from the air syringe.

CHAPTER 4

MATRICES

THE foundation for the two-surfaced or multi-surfaced amalgam restoration is the matrix.

The functions of the matrix band in amalgam restorations are:
1. To reproduce the missing contour of the tooth.
2. To provide an ideal contact area with the adjacent tooth.
3. To prevent cervical overhang of amalgam.
4. To permit adequate condensation of amalgam so as:
   a. To achieve a homogeneous filling with no laminations of successive layers of amalgam;
   b. To reduce the residual mercury content of the amalgam restoration.

Green et al. (1943) have traced the early matrices, which consisted of a piece of metal band wedged in place either by a wooden wedge dipped in sandrac or zinc phosphate cement, to the more modern mechanical matrices and retainers (*Fig.* 75). They are of the opinion, and this is generally supported, that there is no perfect universal matrix holder and retainer.

Phillips et al. (1956) studied five different types of mechanical matrix retainers in relation to their efficiency in restoring the contour of the proximal missing surface of a Class II cavity to be filled with amalgam. In order to ascertain whether any additional advantage could be gained by contouring or wedging these bands, they divided their tests into using the bands: (1) uncontoured and unwedged: (2) uncontoured but wedged; (3) contoured but unwedged; (4) contoured and wedged.

They found that, whether the teeth be ovoid, square, or tapered, wedging is essential to avoid gross cervical overhang of amalgam. They also found that in ovoid and square type teeth, contouring the band in addition was needed to produce the best results, although wedging was the more important factor. However, in the tapering type tooth, contouring the band had little advantage.

Choice of Band

The band replacing the missing contour of the tooth should be 0·0015–0·002 in thick (0·04 mm–0·05 mm). This will allow adequate thinness of metal to permit burnishing and contouring of the proximal portion of the band, and ensure a good contact between the finished restoration and the adjacent tooth, while at the same time being able to withstand condensing pressures without splitting or tearing. A suitable band is chosen so that it extends from just below the cavo-gingival line angle of the cavity to just above the level of the marginal ridge of the adjacent tooth. If the width of the band is insufficient, there is either a gingival space where the amalgam is condensed out of the box of the cavity, or, if properly placed gingivally, amalgam will be condensed between the band and the adjacent tooth when the marginal ridge area is being condensed (*Fig.* 76). If the band is too wide, it is difficult to contour and

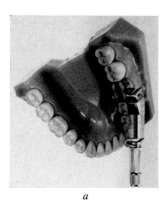

a

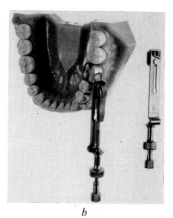

b

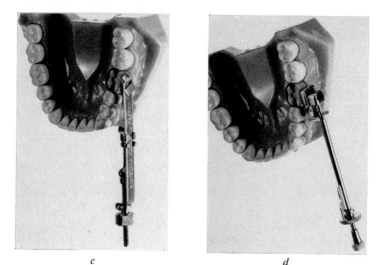

c   *d*

Fig. 75. Types of matrix bands and retainers: *a*, Tofflemire junior retainer; *b*, Dentatus Mec-N matrix holder, accredited to P. Nystrom; *c*, Siqueland retainer; *d*, Bonnalie matrix retainer.

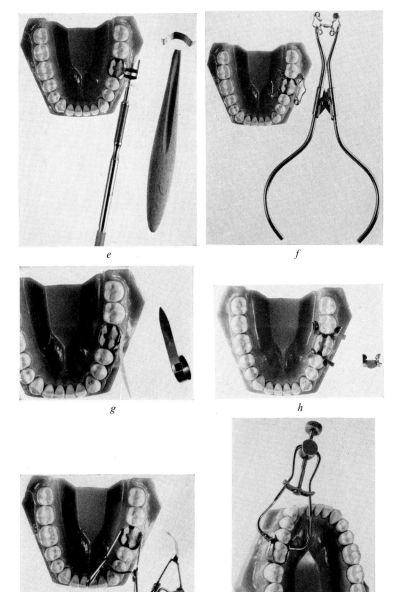

e, Lennox matrix outfit 3L; *f*, Walser matrices; *g*, Dr Levett's matrices; *h*, Neos cervix matrices; *i*, Dr Endres' apis matrix retainer; *j*, Ivory No. 1 matrix retainer.

burnish the band adequately, and this invariably results in too high a contact area. In addition, there is a tendency for a too wide band to be driven down into the periodontal tissues.

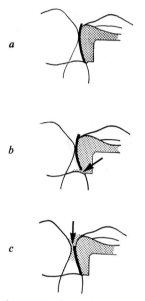

Fig. 76. Correct placement of matrix band: *a*, Band extends correctly from above contact point to gingival crevice; *b*, Insufficient gingival extension of band with consequent escape of amalgam; *c*, Insufficient occlusal extension of band with consequent packing of amalgam through contact area.

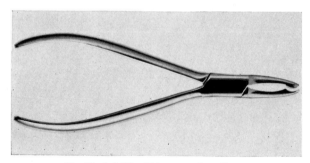

Fig. 77. Ash No. 114 contouring pliers.

Contouring of Band

The band must be contoured in two directions. First, the natural vertical contour of the missing proximal surface of the tooth from the gingival margin up to and including the contact area is copied with contouring pliers (*Fig.* 77). Second, the buccolingual contour of the missing proximal surface is copied with the pliers. There should be no serrations in the beaks of the pliers, otherwise the band will be marked, and these identations can be transferred to the amalgam surface. The use of an uncontoured band fixed to the tooth with a mechanical retainer results in a proximal amalgam wall, which is straight from the gingival margin to its extremity at the marginal ridge. This results in the restoration meeting the adjacent tooth with too high and too pointed a contact point.

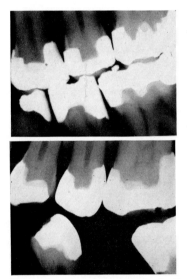

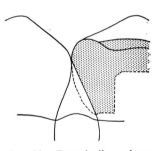

Fig. 79. Dotted line shows additional bulk of amalgam gained by contouring band.

Fig. 78. Comparison of badly contoured and correctly contoured restorations.

Through wear, this type of restoration soon loses its effectiveness (*Fig.* 78), and the resultant harmful effect on the supporting periodontal tissues and the possible subsequent decay of the approximating non-carious surface should be noted.

However, by careful contouring, not only can the correct placement of the contact area be achieved, and the integrity of the gingival tissue be maintained, but there is the added advantage of an increase in amalgam bulk, which will increase the strength of the restoration (*Fig.* 79).

Wedging the Band

After the cavity has been correctly prepared, all the cavo-surface line angles are easily accessible with the cavo-gingival line angle being approached through the cavity. Once, however, the cavity is filled, it is only the cavo-gingival line angle which is not easily accessible to allow carving and polishing instruments to provide a smooth amalgam-enamel junction. Thus, to prevent gingival excess of amalgam remaining permanently, as its removal is difficult, care must be taken to prevent its occurrence.

The effect of amalgam as an exciting cause of periodontal disease has been discussed previously, but, in addition, Castaldi et al. (1957) have pointed out that analyses of residual mercury content in Class II amalgam restorations was higher in proximo-gingival areas than in the bulk of the restoration, and even higher in the flash of the gingival amalgam overhang, if present. The critical importance of a low residual mercury content will be discussed later, but suffice it to say that adequate provision must be made to prevent amalgam flash at the cavo-gingival line angle.

Several matrix bands and retainers have been developed to compensate for the cervical constriction of the teeth. The Ivory No. 1 and the Bonnalie, which are popular matrix retainers in English dental schools, utilize bands which are crescent-shaped, the shorter edge being the gingival edge. By varying the concavity of this gingival edge, the adaptation to the gingival constriction can be varied. The Siqueland, by means of an adjustable toggle, claims adequate adjustable gingival constriction of an unshaped band, while providing adequate divergency occlusally for burnishing a contact area. These bands are difficult to contour, although very easy to apply to the tooth. The Tofflemire makes use of shaped bands as well as a fixed, angulated, retaining slot to provide gingival constriction (*see Fig. 75*).

Nevertheless, in order to ensure tight adaptation of the band at the cavo-gingival line angle, and support it there under correct condensing pressures, an unyielding wedge must be used. Markley (1951) considers that the wedge has the additional task of separating the teeth slightly, in order to compensate for the thickness of the matrix band, and so give a tight contact in the finished restoration. Boyde and Knight (1972) have demonstrated by scanning electron microscope studies that excessively tightening a band to provide a tight fit can produce compression fractures of the enamel at the cavity margins. The use of a proper wedging technique will provide a tight fit of the band at the cavo-gingival line angle without the need to excessively tighten the band and a slight excess of amalgam at the embrasure cavo-surface line angles can be easily removed by subsequent surface finishing techniques.

Various commercial wedges have been produced in celluloid and silver, as well as wood (*Fig. 80*). Since the interproximal space and the amount of curvature of the proximal contour of the tooth varies, stock wedges are not always ideal. Successful wedges are best prepared for each individual restoration, and can be cut from hickory wood sticks or wooden tongue spatulae. The practice of plugging the interdental space with one or more soft wood points, rather like the lateral condensation technique of gutta-percha points in root-canal therapy, is to be discouraged, since this tends to interfere with the contour of the band by actually denting it into the cavity (*Fig.* 81). Kantorowicz (1957) has stressed the importance of preparing the wedge with a triangular form in cross-section, the base resting on the

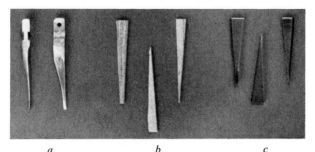

a   *b*   *c*

Fig 80. Types of stock wedges: *a*, Silver wedges; *b*, Wooden wedges; *c*, Plastic wedges.

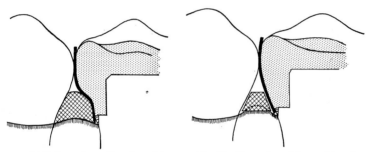

Fig. 81. Indentation of band resulting from excessive wedging.

Fig. 82. Correct wedging of band. A wide base to the wedge will prevent its rotation.

gingival tissues and the sides of the triangle being contoured to follow the contour of the approximating teeth. The apex of the triangle is cut flat or left sharp, depending on the amount of inter-proximal space (*Fig.* 82). He points out that wedges which are rectangular in cross-section, while initially satisfactory, can, during the condensation of amalgam, rotate and so become functionless.

As a guide to the correct placement of matrices, the technique which can be adopted in various instances will be outlined:

63

TECHNIQUE FOR RESTORING A CLASS II CAVITY WITH ONE PROXIMAL WALL MISSING, USING AN IVORY No. 1 RETAINER AND MATRIX BAND

1. *Select Band.* A band which is completely smooth is used. The need for choosing a band which extends from just below the cavo-gingival line angle to just above the marginal ridge of the adjacent tooth has already been stressed. Modification in height can be made with scissors, but care must be taken to smooth any turned or roughened surfaces which may result, otherwise the amalgam restoration can be damaged when the band is removed.

2. *Try the band and retainer on the tooth,* and select the holes in the band into which the jaws of the retainer will fit. These jaws should touch the tooth gingivally to the maximum curvature of the tooth and just beyond the angle of the embrasure, away from the proximal box, so that on tightening the band the jaws slide down an inclined plane, so fixing and tightening the band.

3. *Contour the Band.* The band is then removed and contoured in an occlusogingival and buccolingual direction with contouring pliers.

4. *Fix the Band to the Tooth.* If the proximal box of the cavity is very wide, excessive tightening of the band will tend to draw the band away from the adjacent tooth, and also spoil the prepared contouring. In this case, it is better to slacken the band, and, after wedging and burnishing it, use softened modelling composition to support the band and assist in fixing the matrix retainer.

5. *Wedge the Band.*

6. *Burnish the Contact Area* against the adjacent tooth with a ball-ended burnisher.

The advantage of this type of band and retainer is the ease with which it can be removed without the risk of damage to the contact area and the marginal ridge of the amalgam restoration.

The wedge is first removed, and the retainer is released and removed from the mouth. The band can then be bent back against the adjacent tooth and removed in an occlusolingual or occluso-buccal direction.

TECHNIQUE FOR RESTORING A CLASS II CAVITY WITH MORE THAN ONE WALL MISSING OR A CLASS I CAVITY WITH A BUCCAL OR LINGUAL EXTENSION

In this type of restoration a continuous band has to be used, and this can be fixed to the tooth with a retainer such as the Bonnalie, Siqueland, or Tofflemire retainer. Brown (1955) also described the T-band, similar to Dr Levett's matrix (*Fig.* 83), which can be fixed to the tooth without any retainer.

The Siqueland is the only retainer which cannot be released from the band in the mouth. The result is that the band has to be withdrawn occlusally, with the increased risk of damage to the contact area and marginal ridges of the restoration.

1. *Select Band.* Note should be taken of the height of the band, and also the amount of curvature required to compensate for the cervical constriction of the tooth. Any modification can again be made with scissors.

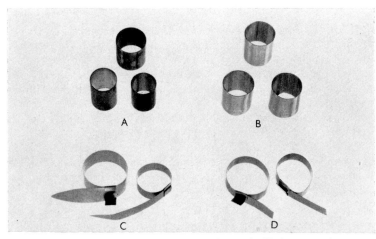

Fig. 83. Bands which can remain on the tooth till the restoration has become sufficiently strong to be left unsupported: A, Copper bands; B, Aluminium bands; C, Dr Levett's matrices; D, T-bands.

2. *Fix the band to the retainer* to be used, and try the band on the tooth. The areas on the band which have to be contoured should be marked lightly with a probe, and the band is removed.

3. *Contour the band* with pliers, as previously described.

4. *Replace the band in the retainer*, and fix it to the tooth by tightening the retainer.

5. *Wedge the band*, as described previously.

6. *Burnish the contact area* against the adjacent tooth with a ball-ended burnisher.

7. *Additional support* can be obtained with softened modelling composition.

After the initial set of the amalgam, the wedge is removed and the retainer is released from the band. One end of the band is bent distally and removed in an occlusobuccal or occlusolingual direction, depending on which side of the tooth the retainer was fixed. The retainer is usually fixed to the band on the buccal side of the tooth, so as to be in the buccal sulcus. Occasionally, however, it is necessary or more convenient to attach the retainer on the lingual side of the tooth. The two ends of the band are then brought mesially and the band is removed, again in an occlusobuccal or occlusolingual direction.

TECHNIQUE FOR RESTORING LARGE CLASS V OR MARKEDLY CONVEX CLASS V CAVITIES WHERE CONDENSING PROCEDURES WOULD TEND TO DRIVE THE AMALGAM OUT OF THE CAVITY

1. *Select a continuous band* and retainer where the retainer can be applied to the lingual or buccal side of the tooth; that is, on the side of the tooth opposite to the cavity.

The band should be tried on the tooth to ensure that the retainer can adequately hold it in place. Mark the outline of the cavity on the band with a probe.

2. *Remove the band* and cut a window in the band slightly smaller than the outline of the cavity.

3. *Reapply the band and retainer* and ensure that all the margins of the cavity are covered by the band, and that there is an adequate window for the condensing instrument to reach all parts of the cavity.

TECHNIQUE FOR RESTORING EXTENSIVE CAVITIES WHERE IT IS ADVISABLE TO LEAVE THE MATRIX BAND IN PLACE UNTIL THE AMALGAM HAS REACHED A SUFFICIENT STRENGTH TO BE LEFT UNSUPPORTED

In extensive cavities, where cusps are having to be restored in amalgam and retention is aided with dentine pins, it is often advisable to leave the band in place until the compressive strength of the amalgam has nearly reached its maximum. In these circumstances the seamless copper or nickel bands or the T-band are used, which require no retainer (*Fig.* 83).

The technique consists of selecting a band which just fits the tooth, and contouring the gingival and occlusal margins with scissors and stones so that it extends to just below the gingival floor of the cavity without damaging any gingival tissue. Occlusally, the band is trimmed, so that it does not interfere with the occlusion.

The band is annealed and contoured to copy the proposed contour of the restoration. The contact area is thinned with stones on the outside of the band, and the band is burnished against the adjacent tooth. A wedge is placed where necessary and the band is supported with composition. Condensation of amalgam against an unsupported annealed band results in buckling of the band.

If the bite will allow, the band can be burnished on to a natural cusp, if present, or turned on to the marginal ridge of the adjacent tooth. This will prevent any risk of gingival damage due to the downward drift of the band during chewing.

Only the wedge and composition are removed after carving the amalgam. Removal of the band is left till the next visit and is achieved by cutting along the buccal or lingual side of the band with a fissure burr.

CHAPTER 5

SILVER AMALGAM MANIPULATION

IT is not only cavity preparation, whether aided or not with auxiliary retention, that influences the strength of the amalgam restoration. The handling or manipulation of the alloy and mercury can greatly influence the strength of the filling.

Following the advent of the A.D.A. Specification No. 1 in 1930, inferior amalgam alloys have now virtually disappeared from the dental market. Failure of an amalgam restoration, therefore, can no longer be attributed to a poor material. However, all alloys which are certified by the British, U.S.A. and Australian Bureaux of Standards are not the same in their management, and the dental practitioner must have a knowledge of the manipulative procedures which will achieve the best physical properties of the alloy chosen. A careful manipulative procedure with amalgam, closely following the manufacturer's instructions, will ensure that the highest standards are achieved and maintained.

CHOICE OF ALLOY

In the choice of an alloy, the factors that will be considered are the alloy composition, the particle shape, particle size, the speed of set, whether to use a pre-amalgamated or standard alloy and whether to use a zinc-containing or zinc-free alloy.

Alloy Composition

The generally accepted specifications for amalgam alloy require the composition of the constituent metals to be 65 per cent minimum silver, 29 per cent maximum tin, 6 per cent maximum copper and 2 per cent maximum zinc. In addition by adding up to 3 per cent maximum mercury, alloys can be more readily amalgamated with mercury at the trituration stage, and are termed 'pre-amalgamated alloys'.

Innes and Youdelis (1963) have shown that, by blending a silver–copper eutectic alloy with the silver–tin alloy, considerable improvement in the physical properties of the resultant amalgam is obtained. More recently, Acharya et al. (1973) have shown some improvement in the physical properties of amalgam by the admixing of copper amalgam with silver amalgam alloys. Essentially these systems claim to reduce the amount of weaker tin/mercury phase in the final set amalgam with its resultant improvement in corrosion resistance, and compressive and edge strengths. The alloy system developed by Innes and Youdelis is now commercially available under the name of Dispersalloy and the main clinical advantages claimed for it over the more conventional alloys are its greater resistance to tarnish and corrosion and its improved edge strength with consequent reduction in marginal failure leading to 'ditching'. However, since it is possible by careful manipulative techniques to minimize the amount of the weaker tin/mercury phase using conventional alloys, the practitioner may well be justified in awaiting the results of longer term clinical trials before changing to the more expensive new alloy systems.

In an attempt to improve the resistance to marginal recurrent caries Jerman (1970) found that, by adding 1·5 per cent stannous fluoride to the alloy, there was an increased fluoride content of the enamel adjacent to the restoration with an associated reduction in enamel solubility. Although the anticariogenic property of a silicate cement restoration has been shown, there is evidence that there is continued leaching of the fluoride from the silicate cement but this has not been demonstrated in the case of the set amalgam restoration. Stoner et al. (1971) have in addition shown a deterioration to corrosion resistance in alloys containing stannous or sodium fluoride.

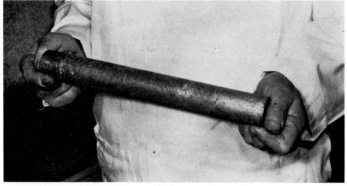

Fig. 84. Ingot of silver amalgam alloy.

Particle Shape

In the manufacture of silver amalgam alloy, the main constituents, namely, silver, tin, copper and zinc, are melted and cast to form an ingot of the alloy (*Fig.* 84). This ingot is then comminuted into filings by turning on a lathe (*Fig.* 85). These filings are subsequently broken down in size in a ball mill. A method of sieving ensures that the chosen size of particle is achieved, the larger particles being returned to the ball mill for further milling. These resultant lathe cut particles are irregular flake-shaped and although similar in size as a result of sieving are not necessarily similar in shape.

Demaree and Taylor (1962) used particles in the form of spheres made by the atomization of the molten alloy, which were later graded into various sizes by sieving. This eliminated the effect of shape on the various particle sizes. They showed that particle sizes of 15–50 µ gave the most desirable properties in relation to compressive strength, dimensional change on setting, and residual mercury content. They suggest that the spherical particle alloy is more advantageous than the conventional lathe-cut alloy in that it is possible to control the physical properties of the amalgam by suitable

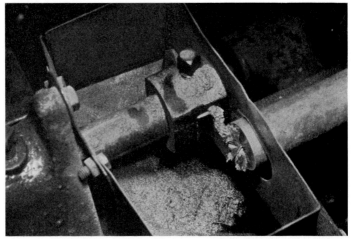

Fig. 85. Production of lathe-cut particles from ingot.

blending of the various spherical particle sizes. Apart from better physical properties, Demaree and Taylor also claim that its production is easier than the conventional alloy manufacturing process and is also less sensitive to manipulative variables, such as further breaking up during trituration, since it is more likely that the particles will roll and not fracture.

Koran and Asgar (1967) in a comparison of dental amalgams made from spherical and lathe-cut alloys claimed superior 1-hour compressive strengths, final compressive strengths and tensile strengths for the spherical particle alloys. They recommended using 10–37 µ graded spherical particle sizes.

Basker and Wilson (1971), however, considered that spherical particle alloys are stronger than the conventional materials only during the very early stages of hardening. Wing (1966), in addition, has shown that spherical particle amalgam alloys adapt less well to the cavity wall than well condensed lathe-cut alloys. One of the main clinical advantages in using spherical alloy particles is the increased plasticity of the mix with mercury which facilitates condensation around pins used for auxiliary retention. This facility, coupled with the improved 1-hour compressive strength, is an indication for its use in multi-pinned amalgam restorations. Care must be taken to wedge and support the matrix band adequately to prevent gingival amalgam excess resulting from the condensation of this more plastic spherical alloy amalgam.

Particle Size

In recent years there has been a trend towards the use of alloys that have a smaller particle size. Since the restoration is composed of particles of the original alloy (silver/tin phase) surrounded by mercury, silver/mercury and tin/mercury phases, the original particle size alters the character of the finished, carved, and polished surface. Crowell and Phillips (1951) have shown that, when all other manufacturing variables are carefully controlled, there is a definite relationship between strength and particle size. The smaller the particle the higher the 1-hour and 24-hour strengths.

Jarabak (1942) has done research on the relationship of other properties of amalgam to particle size. His conclusions in respect of a reduction in particle size were that expansion decreases, there is a lessening of the effect of trituration on dimensional change, and the effect of condensation on dimensional change becomes less apparent. Further, he showed that there was a greater sensitivity to dimensional change in the coarser particle sizes for controlled trituration and condensation.

Skinner and Phillips (1960) support the use of smaller size particles because the triturated small grained alloy is more easily adapted to the cavity walls. In addition the carved surface of a small grained amalgam is much less pitted and consequently more easily polished owing to the tendency for larger particles to be pulled out of the matrix while carving. Mahler et al. (1973) have shown that excessively small or microcut alloy particles produce a faster setting amalgam restoration, having less plasticity than that produced by the slightly larger or fine-cut alloy particles and, in addition, has relatively poorer marginal strength. The consensus of opinion is in favour of the use of fine-cut amalgam alloy particles.

Speed of Set

The setting time of an alloy is accelerated by increasing the silver content. Whilst the minimum content of silver is 65 per cent in the

A.D.A. Specification, some very rapid setting alloys have a silver content of over 70 per cent.

Micro-cut amalgam alloys also have a faster speed of set, because of the greater number of centres of crystallization present.

In using faster setting alloys, care should be taken to condense quickly, and in large cavities more than one fresh mix of the alloy and mercury may have to be used, rather than one large mix, otherwise crystallization will have started in the uncondensed amalgam before it is placed in the cavity, and the resultant filling will have poor strength.

A fast-setting alloy has the advantage that it reduces the time the patient is in the chair. In addition, some dentists use a fast-setting alloy when they are forced to fill approximal cavities at one appointment. This procedure is normally not justified, since there is the risk when filling the second cavity of damaging the marginal ridge and contact area of the previously inserted approximal filling. Even if the practitioner is very careful, the resultant component forces of condensation pressures exerted when packing the amalgam in the contact area of the second cavity will tend to draw mercury to this surface in the previously filled cavity. This will invite pitting and corrosion in this area. It is doubtful if there will be actual amalgamation of the two fillings if they are filled separately at the same appointment.

The main disadvantage of too rapid a setting amalgam is the rapid crystallization, which limits the removal of mercury from successive condensed portions of amalgam already in the cavity. In this regard, Phillips and Boyd (1947) have shown that, where there is an increase of residual mercury in the amalgam restoration, there is a reduction in the crushing strength, an increase in flow, and a reduction in the resistance of the restoration to tarnish and corrosion. They are, however, of the opinion that, if it is possible to express excess mercury by condensation, then the use of quick-setting alloys increases the initial hardness of the filling considerably.

Pre-amalgamated Amalgam Alloys

Pre-amalgamated lathe-cut or spherical alloys are produced by treating the alloy particles with mercuric chloride thus coating the particles with mercury. The A.D.A. specification for silver amalgam alloy allows for a maximum content of 3 per cent mercury though 1–2 per cent is more common in proprietary pre-amalgamated alloys. It has been shown that by using pre-amalgamated alloys a reduced ratio of mercury to alloy can be used which amalgamates very readily. Jorgensen et al. (1964) claim that by using pre-amalgamated alloys a residual mercury content below 40 per cent can be obtained.

However, Staheli and von Fraunhofer (1971) have shown that pre-amalgamated alloys offer no advantage over non pre-amalgamated alloys with regard to microhardness and compressive strength properties. The clinical advantages of using pre-amalgamated alloys appear to be the ease and speed of trituration with mercury and the ease of condensation of the resultant more plastic mix. In addition, Forsten (1969) has shown that pre-amalgamated zinc-containing alloys show less delayed expansion when contaminated with moisture than non-pre-amalgamated alloys. The suggested reason for this is that when the pre-amalgamation process of treating the alloy particles with mercuric chloride in a weak acid is followed by washing away the excess mercuric chloride with sulphuric acid, zinc on the surface of the alloy particles is dissolved and removed. Thus, there is less zinc available for the related deleterious effects of moisture contamination.

Non-zinc Alloys

It is known that the excessive delayed expansion of amalgam resulting from moisture contamination is due to the presence of zinc in the alloy, which dissociates the water, liberating hydrogen gas. This fact has led to interest in using non-zinc alloys, since it has been shown that if zinc is excluded from the alloy, this excessive delayed expansion does not take place.

Van Gunst and Hertog (1957) have shown that, if the zinc content of the alloy is less than 0·01 per cent, there is no delayed expansion when contaminated with moisture. However, the presence of 0·06 per cent of zinc in the alloy will produce the maximum delayed expansion that can be attributed to the moisture contamination of zinc-containing alloys. The manufacturers' claim that an alloy has only a trace of zinc may be meaningless, as that trace of 0·06 per cent will produce the maximum delayed expansion, which they found to be in the range of $2\frac{1}{2}$–6 per cent.

Phillips et al. (1954) have tested non-zinc alloys, and found that they have essentially the same physical properties of zinc-containing alloys, although the zinc-free alloys are considered to tarnish more rapidly. However, Phillips (1973) reports that clinical studies do not support these laboratory findings and show increased marginal deterioration in the case of zinc-free alloys. Forsten (1969) found that moisture contamination of zinc-free amalgams did in fact produce a 10 per cent reduction in compressive strengths and a 5 per cent decrease in transverse strengths compared with the uncontaminated zinc free amalgams. This he considered was due to the mechanical factor of the liquid reducing the cohesion of the amalgam during condensation.

Sweeney (1941) has shown that, when non-zinc alloys are contaminated with water, the resultant restoration has a pitted surface, which is much more easily corroded.

It is therefore clear that since zinc-free alloys should be protected from moisture contamination, the better properties such as surface lustre obtained from zinc-containing alloys are to be preferred. Whenever moisture contamination cannot be prevented by adequate isolation of the tooth a zinc-free alloy should be used.

Choice of Mercury

Mercury complying with the requirements of the British and U.S.A. Pharmacopoeia, or the A.D.A. Specification No. 6, should be used. The most recent British Standards Specification for Dental Mercury is B.S. 4227 and was published in 1967. The mercury must contain less than 0·02 per cent by mass, non-volatile residue and there must be no visible surface contamination. The silvery surface brightness is easily lost when mercury is slightly contaminated and, unless the mercury has a mirror-like surface, it should not be used.

Tarnished mercury, as distinct from contaminated mercury coming out from wet mixes after trituration with amalgam alloy, can be cleaned by the dental nurse. The tarnished mercury is passed through a pin-prick hole in filter-paper held in a glass filter-funnel and allowed to drop into a carefully cleaned glass dispenser. Alternatively, the tarnished mercury can be passed through clean chamois skin to restore its previous brightness. Mercury contaminated by the metals of the amalgam alloy can only be purified by distillation procedures. The use of such contaminated mercury for further trituration with amalgam alloy will delay amalgamation.

Perhaps the most powerful criticism levelled against amalgam, which influenced its slow general adoption in the early days as a filling material, has been the claim that it caused mercury poisoning. It is true that filling teeth with amalgam does imply a certain exposure of the patient to mercury. Since mercury will vaporize at mouth temperature, this exposure is mainly caused by the evolution of mercury vapour during the insertion of the filling. However, the vapour pressure at this temperature would only allow an infinitesimal amount of mercury to vaporize. Swallowing of fresh amalgam may play a part while the continuous abrasion of the filling once completed seems to add very little to the total exposure.

Chan and Svare (1972) in their studies have shown that mercury vapour is greatest at the margins of the restoration, indicating that there is probably a higher mercury content in these areas. In addition, they have shown that there is no difference in the amount of mercury vapour given off whether the surface of the amalgam is burnished or carved. This emission of mercury vapour in fact diminished with time and was undetectable after five days.

Frykholm (1957) has reported that there is no clinical or experimental evidence to indicate that there is enough mercury or amalgam absorbed by the patient, either during insertion or during the life of the restoration, to give rise to systemic mercury poisoning. However, he has reported several cases of allergic reaction to mercury, and considers that the cases of systemic mercury poisoning associated with amalgam fillings, which were reported in the early literature, were in reality cases of allergy. Further, the majority of the cases of allergy showed only temporary symptoms, which disappeared once the mercury in the restoration had combined in stable phases.

Hitchin and Hall (1963) reported a case of allergic reaction, traced in fact to the silver in the restoration and not to any of the other constituents of silver amalgam.

While these cases of allergy are very rare when one considers the billions of amalgam fillings inserted, the dentist must take note of their possibility, and, as far as the patients are concerned, alternative restorative materials can be used. Shovelton (1968) has reported the successful treatment of a patient with mercury allergy using amalgam as a restorative material by the prophylactic administration of antihistamine tablets combined with a careful insertion of the amalgam into the cavity so that no excess falls into the mouth. Subsequently he coated the filling with varnish.

The dental surgeon and his staff, however, are not in such limited contact with mercury. They handle it every day for many years and it may in fact, because of the risk of sensitization, prove a hazard to health, especially when working in confined, poorly ventilated surgeries where the procedure is to wring out excess mercury from wet mixes on to the floor, spill mercury when pouring into small dispensers from bulk buying jars, or indulge in the bad practice of mulling the triturated mix in the hand.

Cook and Yates (1969) reported on a fatality involving a dental surgery assistant with a history of working in a dental surgery for 20 years. The assistant died from acute renal failure attributed to mercury intoxication. The histological examination of the kidneys using staining techniques to demonstrate mercury showed the generalized presence of mercury. Although this case is considered to be unique, it has served as a warning that the dental practitioner and his surgery assistants are exposed to the hazard of mercury intoxication and that every effort should be made to ensure a safe working environment.

Many studies have been done on the concentration of mercury

vapour in dental surgeries, and clearly show that the safe industrial setting for mercury in the atmosphere is exceeded in some surgeries. The safe industrial setting for mercury in the atmosphere is 0·05 milligrams of mercury per cubic metre of air breathed in an 8-hour day over a 40-hour week and is known as the T.L.V., the threshold limit value. Vapour concentrations lower than this T.L.V. are not considered to produce any symptoms and such contamination as occurs is easily cleared by the kidneys from the blood. However, vapour concentrations above a T.L.V. of 0·05 mg/m³ produced symptoms of mercuralism in some workers. As the symptoms appear the urine level of mercury decreases, indicating a reduced ability of the kidneys to excrete the mercury. It is for this reason that urine levels are not a good guide to mercury intoxication.

It should suffice to say that care must be exercised when handling mercury and the dental practitioner must be responsible for establishing a high standard of mercury hygiene in his surgery. All mercury and waste amalgam should be kept in tightly sealed containers. Spilled mercury should be cleared up immediately, and that in inaccessible crevices should be treated with flowers of sulphur. The alloy-mercury mix should never be handled for, apart from contaminating the amalgam with perspiration, it can produce allergic reactions in sensitized people.

Proportioning Mercury to Alloy

No one factor has a more profound influence on the final properties of amalgam than the eventual mercury content of the amalgam restoration. The original work done in the relation of strength of amalgam to mercury content was carried out by Gray (1919).

The factors which influence the amount of mercury left in the final restoration are:

1. The original mercury/alloy ratio;
2. The amount of trituration;
3. The amount of excess mercury expressed prior to condensation;
4. The duration and pressure of condensation.

With regard to mercury/alloy ratio, Phillips and Swartz (1949) have shown that, regardless of the amount squeezed away in the squeeze-cloth or removed by condensation, the more mercury used in the original mix the greater is the amount that will remain in the restoration. Phillips and Boyd (1947) have shown by chemical analysis that, as the mercury/alloy ratio is increased, the percentage of residual mercury also increases proportionally, and they found that, for each additional 15 per cent of mercury used in the original mix, there is an average increase of 1–1·5 per cent residual mercury.

Analyses of clinical amalgam restorations show a wide variation in residual mercury content, reaching as high as 70 per cent. Swartz and Phillips (1956) have shown that the mercury content of amalgam restorations is invariably greater at the marginal areas, usually by 2–3 per cent. Their findings were that compressive strengths were not altered appreciably by fluctuations in residual mercury content between 50 per cent and 55 per cent, but that there was a serious loss of strength when the mercury content exceeded 55 per cent. For example, one commercial alloy tested by them had a compressive strength of 40,000 lb/sq in (276 MN/m²) at a residual mercury content of 55 per cent; this dropped to only 18,000 lb/sq in (124 MN/m²) when the mercury content rose to 59 per cent. A strength of 18,000 lb/sq in (124 MN/m²) would not be adequate to withstand normal biting stresses.

In a clinical investigation of the relation of mercury to the amalgam restoration, where fillings of varying known residual mercury content were inserted, Nadal et al. (1961) have shown that marginal deterioration and surface roughness are also increased when the residual mercury content goes above 55 per cent. It should be noted that an amalgam with a residual mercury content of less than 45 per cent, while by laboratory tests producing a restoration having a slightly higher compressive strength, will, in fact, provide too dry a mix for clinical use. On condensation into a cavity it will result in successive layers of amalgam not amalgamating with each other, and so lead to a laminated restoration with weaker properties. These results emphasize the need to maintain an accurate control of the mercury/alloy ratio, and they recommend that a standardized procedure, such as the Eames' minimal mercury technique, should be followed.

Eames (1959) has fathered the change from the generally accepted technique of using a mercury/alloy ratio of 8 : 5 by weight triturated in a pestle and mortar, rubber thumbstall or mechanical amalgamator, to using a mercury/alloy ratio of 1 : 1, which can only be triturated in a mechanical amalgamator. Using this technique, there is no need to express mercury after trituration, or to use heavy condensing pressures to reduce the residual mercury content of the restoration, since one is commencing with a mercury content below the critical 55 per cent residual mercury content.

Jorgensen et al. (1966), however, have shown that by increasing the initial mercury/alloy ratio to produce a wet mix with a mercury content as high as 65 per cent it is possible subsequently to express the excess mercury to produce a residual mercury content to below 50 per cent. They claim that such a prepared amalgam has less porosity and greater crushing strength than amalgam prepared from an initial mercury/alloy ratio of 1 : 1. Eames et al. (1961) recognize

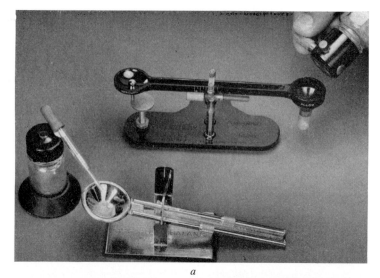

a

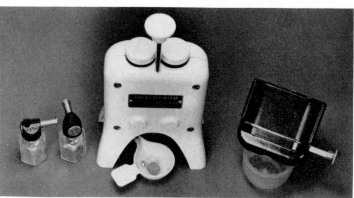

b

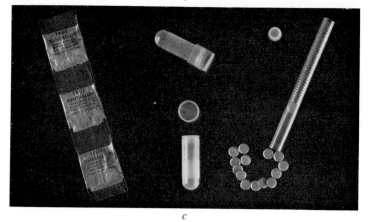

c

the advantages of a more plastic mix and advise when using a 1 : 1 ratio of mercury and alloy to over-triturate slightly.

The problem then arises which is the best method of dispensing the correct proportions of mercury to alloy (*Fig.* 86). Sweeney (1944) is of the opinion that the proportion of mercury to alloy should be weighed out according to the manufacturer's instructions. He suggests storing the weighed out alloy in clear gelatin capsules, and the mercury in coloured gelatin capsules. The more common method of dispensing alloy and mercury is the automatic release type of dispenser, which proportions the alloy and mercury volumetrically. However, it must be stressed that, if automatic dispensers are used in a practice where alloys of varying particle sizes are employed, then the dispenser must be adjusted accordingly. If this is not done, since a lesser weight of larger grained alloy will occupy a given volume of well in a dispenser compared with a smaller grained alloy, the desired proportions of a larger grained alloy to mercury will be incorrect if the dispenser has been unadjusted from use with a smaller grained alloy. Mechanical instruments have now been developed which will, in the one appliance, dispense and triturate the alloy and mercury (*Fig.* 87). It is good practice to check from time to time by weighing that the volume dispenser is working correctly.

Ryge et al. (1958) have analysed the accuracy of twelve different methods of obtaining the desired proportions of alloy to mercury. They have shown that there is a marked difference in the degree of accuracy of dispensing, and, apart from the prepacked alloy, no dispensing method gave consistent successive quantities of alloy. They showed that the best method of obtaining an accurate mercury/alloy ratio was to use predispensed alloy produced by the manufacturer, together with a good mercury volume dispenser. The mercury dispenser can be adjusted to give the desired ratio with a given alloy, provided that the dispenser is held vertically, so that the mercury can fall easily, and that the dispenser is not allowed to get more than a third empty. The predispensed alloy can either be obtained in sigren (6 gr) cellophane envelopes or as condensed pellets. Preportioned disposable capsules (*Fig.* 86c) have also been developed which contain the desired ratio of alloy and mercury separated by a disc which is ruptured prior to trituration.

Fig. 86. Examples of proportioning alloy and mercury: *a*, By weight —Crescent and Ash balances; *b*, By volume—Baker proportioner, Amalganom (Heimerle & Meule), S.S. White proportioner; *c*, Predispensed—S.S. White sigrens, Amalcap capsules with mercury in cap, Aristalloy tablets.

Since a proper ratio of mercury to alloy is so important to produce a strong restoration, it behoves every dentist to see that either he or his nurse uses the correct, specified proportions.

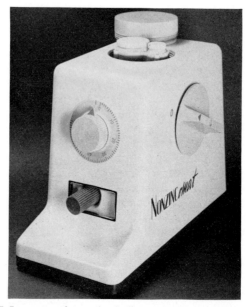

Fig. 87. Instrument for mechanically proportioning and triturating alloy and mercury. The mercury/alloy ratio is controlled by a screw on the hidden side of the appliance.

Preparation of Amalgam for Insertion into the Cavity

TRITURATION: The purpose of trituration is to bring the particles of alloy into contact with the mercury. If this is not done properly the result is a fast-setting, high expanding amalgam, producing a weaker filling. It has further been shown that, where alloy particles have not come into contact with mercury, either as a result of insufficient mercury in the original mix or under amalgamation, voids are caused in the completed restoration which lead to pitting and corrosion.

With proper amalgamation, the amalgam handles smoothly, the working time is adequate, and the carved and polished surface will be more resistant to deterioration.

Although many operators today consider that the mechanical amalgamator is the most accurate method of trituration, Phillips (1944) has shown that there is no evidence that mechanical trituration produces a mix or restoration that is superior to one produced by a careful hand technique. He does agree, however, that mechanical trituration does tend to standardize the procedure in the average person's hand. With the Eames minimal mercury technique a mechanical amalgamator is essential since excess mercury is not available to lubricate the mass. Nixon and Rowbotham (1971) have also drawn attention to the hazard of mercury leakage during mechanical amalgamation.

The pestle and mortar is the most common hand technique of trituration, and consists of rotating a matched pestle in a mortar, into which the dispensed alloy and mercury has been placed. This hand mixing is continued until a shiny, homogeneous mass is obtained (*Fig.* 88). The time taken to mix a given amount of amalgam adequately depends on the force and speed of mixing, and it is for this reason that the mechanical amalgamator produces a more standardized mix.

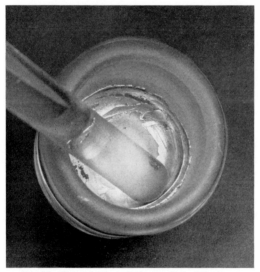

Fig. 88. Correct mix using a pestle and mortar.

Marie Gayler (1934) advocated the amalgamation of alloy and mercury in a rubber thumbstall. This technique has the advantage of not destroying the original particle size of alloy, but a higher mercury/alloy ratio of 9 : 5 is used to obtain amalgamation in 1 minute.

Ambrose (1962) has reported on triturating alloy and mercury, using a pressure amalgamator. This consists of a mechanical device which forces the alloy grains through the mercury in their correct proportions, excess mercury being subsequently expressed in the amalgamator. Nakamura et al. (1961), who tested the physical properties of amalgam mixed by pressure alone, found that the residual mercury content, crushing strength, expansion, and corrosion resistance of this amalgam compared very favourably with amalgam triturated by the more standard techniques.

Over-trituration tends to affect the dimensional change on setting, in as much as the longer the mixing time the less will be the expansion. However, there is no evidence to indicate that the reduced expansion or possible contraction, as detected by laboratory tests, is clinically significant. MacDonald and Phillips (1950) have made observations on clinical restorations placed from over-triturated amalgam, and also with special alloys fabricated to produce excessive contraction. They have failed to show a single instance of open margins or recurrent caries. The restorations placed with the thoroughly amalgamated mix proved superior in terms of surface condition and marginal adaptation. Originally, it was thought that the 'ditched' effect around amalgam restorations (see Fig. 2) was due to the contraction of the amalgam, but this is now considered more likely to be due to:

1. Insufficient extension of the cavity preparation to smooth enamel margins so that weak spurs of amalgam result in pits and fissures at the periphery of the restoration;

2. A bevelled cavo-surface line angle, resulting in the breaking off of the feathered edge of amalgam;

3. Poor condensation techniques, which leave these areas with a high mercury content and consequently a weaker edge strength;

4. The result of breaking off an original feathered edge of amalgam remaining after poor carving and polishing procedures.

Eames et al. (1961) have suggested that, when using a 1 : 1 ratio of alloy and mercury, it is better to over-triturate slightly, and so produce a more plastic mix. This increased plasticity of the amalgam requires less condensing force to unite the successive layers to produce a homogeneous filling, and consequently minimizes the traumatic effect of heavy condensing pressures on the underlying base. Thus, a zinc oxide/eugenol type lining can be used more readily without fear of its destruction under condensing pressures. In addition, Swerdlow and Stanley (1962) claim that pulpal damage can result from heavy condensation pressures, despite the presence of a relatively thick wall of dentine.

The consensus of opinion is certainly that it is better to err on the side of too much than too little trituration.

MOISTURE CONTAMINATION: Healey and Phillips (1949) have claimed that approximately 16 per cent of all failures of amalgam restorations can be attributed to excessive expansion due to moisture contamination. Sweeney (1944) has enumerated the effects of moisture contamination on amalgam restorations as:

82

1. A wet cavity will result in margin leakage by the subsequent dissolving of salivary salts;
2. Incorporation of moisture in the amalgam mass will decrease compressive strength;
3. Moisture will cause excessive expansion of alloys containing zinc.

Phillips et al. (1954) have shown by their experiments that contamination of alloys containing zinc produces a 24 per cent reduction in strength, as compared with that of uncontaminated specimens. Further, that the loss in strength becomes apparent after one month, occurring simultaneously with the delayed expansion reaction. This loss in strength is of clinical significance, and unquestionably increases the possibility of fracture when the restoration is subjected to masticatory stress. Forsten (1969) has shown that contamination of zinc-containing amalgam before trituration produces a 30 per cent lower compressive strength than that contaminated after trituration. He agrees that contamination after trituration results on average in a 25 per cent lower compressive strength than that of uncontaminated amalgam. Forsten has also shown that moisture contamination of zinc-containing amalgams prior to trituration in fact produces greater delayed expansion than that produced after trituration.

It has been previously pointed out that the cause of this delayed excessive expansion is due to the dissociation of the water by the zinc present in the alloy, which liberates hydrogen gas. This expansion not only causes internal voids, with the resultant weakening of the restoration, but also, the expansion, which might be as much as 500 microns per centimetre, causes overhanging margins, which invites stagnation and the possibility of recurrent caries. If the contaminated amalgam is unable to expand outside the cavity, it can lead to excessive intracavity pressure, causing pain and possible fracture of tooth tissue.

Since moisture coming into contact with the surface of a condensed amalgam filling has no deleterious effect, any harmful results of moisture contamination must be attributed to the trituration or condensation stages of manipulation. The practice of mulling, which is really continuing the trituration procedure, should never be done in the palm of the hand, because the amalgam can be contaminated with perspiration. A safe method is to place the triturated amalgam in a piece of rubber dam or fingerstall, and rub to the desired plasticity with finger and thumb.

Research workers, from G. V. Black to the present time, have recommended the isolation of the tooth to be restored with a rubber dam, to prevent contamination of the amalgam during the condensation procedure. Although most general practitioners consider the use of rubber dam an unnecessary chore, adequate isolation of the tooth, possibly with cotton-wool rolls, must be established to prevent moisture contamination of the amalgam.

Insertion of Amalgam into the Cavity

The reasons for careful condensation of amalgam are to reduce the residual mercury content and to ensure that the amalgam reaches all parts of the preparation.

Harvey (1946) and Mosteller (1950) have both set the maximum time limit for safe condensation at 3 minutes. It has been a well-recognized fact that prolonging plasticity by continuing to mull the amalgam beyond its normal initial setting time, or replasticizing it by adding fresh mercury, will seriously reduce its strength. If a larger cavity demands much longer working time for amalgam condensation, the use of multiple mixes will allow the operator to handle new plastic amalgam throughout the condensing procedure, and ensure the building up of a homogeneous restoration. Freshly prepared amalgam has more desirable working properties, since the mercury has not had time to be trapped within the newly crystallized mass, nor are the forming crystals fractured during condensation.

A considerable amount of research has been done to ascertain the best method of packing amalgam into the cavity. Both manual and mechanical techniques have been developed, and they both have certain advantages and shortcomings.

Ryge et al. (1952) have demonstrated that mechanical methods of condensation generally cause the amalgam to harden sooner, and have a higher ultimate compressive strength than those which have been condensed by hand. This is supported by McHugh (1955), who adds that adaptation and microhardness tests at the edges of the specimens demonstrate the better results obtained by mechanical packing techniques.

In addition, the manual pressure needed for condensation with mechanical pluggers is much less than that with the hand condensation technique, so maintaining with less fatigue a constant standard of restoration.

The disadvantages of the mechanical methods of condensation lie in the risk of damaging the enamel margin with the plugger point of the condenser, which is more likely with the mallet type of mechanical condenser. The vibrator type of condenser tends to pool mercury at the periphery of the restoration, with the resultant effects of a higher residual mercury content in this area. This can be overcome by grossly overfilling the cavity and carving the higher mercury content amalgam away (*Fig.* 89). Many patients find that the noise and vibrations produced by mechanical condensation are very much more unpleasant than those of hand condensation. Karlström (1950), in an attempt to overcome this discomfort to the patient, tried to develop an ultrasonic amalgam condenser, the vibrations of which would be imperceptible to the patient. However, these have not been shown to produce a superior restoration to the more standard hand or mechanical techniques. There is, in addition, the possibility of ultrasonic condensation producing a fine mercury aerosol with its attendant hazards.

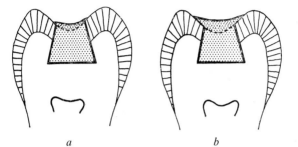

a   *b*

Fig. 89. *a*, Cavities are overfilled to bring free mercury into superficial amalgam excess. Gross excess of amalgam (*b*) is required when using the Dentatus condenser because of the pooling of mercury towards the cavity margins.

It should be noted that the strength of a properly hand-condensed amalgam will provide a restoration that exceeds the requirements of the A.D.A. Specification. In addition, Mizera and Skinner (1961) have shown that, provided the alloy/mercury ratio is below 5 : 6·5, higher 1-hour and 7-day compressive strengths were achieved with hand-condensation methods, as compared with mechanical condensation.

The choice between hand and mechanical condensation seems to be one of personal clinical preference.

HAND CONDENSATION: A good amalgam condensation technique depends on the use of:

1. Small increments of amalgam.
2. Properly designed instruments, to ensure that the amalgam is condensed into all the line angles of the cavity (*Fig.* 90).
3. Heavy condensation pressures.
4. Over-packing the surface of the cavity in order to ensure that the excess mercury which comes to the surface can be carved away. This will leave the final surface of the restoration with as low a residual mercury content as possible.

The technique of adding small quantities of amalgam, condensing each successively, and removing excess plashy material before the next increment is added is probably the most universally followed technique of filling a cavity. If the more conventional mercury/ alloy ratio of 1 : 1·6 (5 : 8) is used, then some excess mercury must be squeezed away in a napkin or chamois after trituration. The squeezed amalgam is then divided into several pieces, the number depending on the size of the cavity. Before inserting the first piece, it is squeezed more vigorously, in order to express as much mercury as possible, commensurate with leaving the amalgam sufficiently plastic to allow adaptation to the cavity walls and cohesion with other increments. Laminations result if over-dry amalgam is used.

When the first portion has been condensed, the successive portions of the divided amalgam are added after first squeezing excess mercury away. It will be noticed that the successive portions require more force to squeeze away mercury. This is because more free mercury

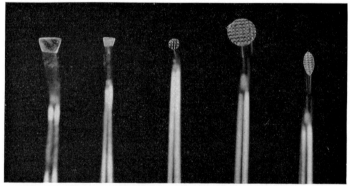

Fig. 90. Hand condensing instruments. From left to right—Ash E, Ash F, 154, 154S, 151.

is reacting with the alloy particles. Some operators prefer to use Chott's pliers to ensure the removal of free mercury; however, care should again be taken not to make the amalgam too dry. Other mechanical devices are available for expressing excess mercury. The 'Amalgamaster' is an instrument using the centrifugal principle of expressing excess mercury. A time dial in seconds controls the amount of mercury extracted from the amalgam mass.

In condensing, the amalgam should be packed on to the gingival or pulpal floors and then against the walls of the cavity, so that the more plashy and weaker amalgam is brought to the centre of the cavity. This will ensure that the residual mercury content of the amalgam in contact with the walls of the cavity will be below the critical 55 per cent level, and so enhance resistance to flow and marginal disintegration.

Care should be taken when condensing with hand instruments to use points that are shaped approximately to the outline of the area being restored (*Fig.* 91). Ramsay (1941) refers to the 'spheroiding' of amalgam at the internal line angles which result if adequately designed instruments are not used (*Fig.* 92). Although small points can be used initially to ensure condensation in the internal line angles of the cavity, their use in condensing successive layers results

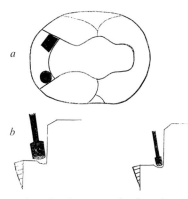

Fig. 91. Necessity of using correctly shaped condensing points. *a*, Advantage of trapezoid point at the sharp internal angles of cavity; *b*, Advantage of a small condensing point in ensuring adequate condensation of amalgam into retention grooves.

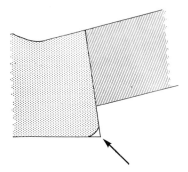

Fig. 92. Arrow indicates 'spheroiding' of amalgam at internal angle as a result of incorrect condensation technique.

in holes being punched into the previously condensed amalgam, rather than uniting the successive increments.

Hatt (1959) has shown that the conventional pen or palm grip of the hand pluggers will allow thrusts of up to 44N(10 lb) but thrusts above 44N(10 lb) are not clinically feasible.

Basker et al. (1973) recommend using a condensing point of 1–2 mm in diameter with a hand thrust of 15 N (3–4 lb) for lathe cut alloys and 8 N (2 lb) for spherical alloys. The previously recommended condensing loads of 36–44 N (8–10 lb) are not clinically feasible.

When using a mercury/alloy ratio of 1 : 1, there is no need to remove mercury with a squeeze cloth, as the residual mercury content commences at 50 per cent. Eames et al. (1961) advocate using a lighter condensing pressure than that in the more conventional techniques, as the object of condensing in this technique is to ensure close adaptation of the amalgam to the cavity, and amalgamation of the successive layers, without necessarily reducing the residual mercury content.

It is good practice, whichever technique is used, to overfill the cavity with amalgam, in order to ensure close adaptation at the cavo-surface line angles, and at the same time bring free mercury up into the superficial amalgam. When the excess amalgam is removed during the carving and finishing procedures, the surface layers of the restoration will have better physical properties as a result of the lower residual mercury content.

MECHANICAL CONDENSATION: The principal advantages of mechanical condensation are: the consistency of standard attained, the reduced dentist fatigue, and the assurance that there is some protection against a premature fracture of the restoration during the first few hours after insertion, because of the increase in initial hardness.

The two most commonly used mechanical condensers are the mallet type and the vibrating type. Condensation is achieved with points held in a contra-angle handpiece worked off the dental engine. There is a selection of condenser points to fit each of these handpieces, and care should be taken to use the points which will ensure close adaptation of the amalgam to the internal detail of the cavity. Successive portions of amalgam can be condensed with the larger points. In the U.S.A. a pneumatic type of condenser, producing a mallet-type thrust, designed by Hollenbach, is popular, as it is equally useful for condensing gold foil.

It should be remembered that the force supplied by the automatic condensers is not in itself enough adequately to condense the amalgam, and additional hand pressure on the handpiece should be applied.

Because of the risk of damage to the enamel prisms at the cavo-surface line angles by the mallet type of condenser, the vibrator type of mechanical condenser is to be preferred.

The Bergendal technique (after the originator of the Dentatus Amalgam Vibrator—*Fig.* 93) consisted of vibrating a small amount of amalgam into the internal aspects of the cavity with a small condensing point, and then following this with a large excess of amalgam covered with a celluloid strip, vibrated home with a large condensing point. This is not a particularly good technique, as vibration is kept to a few seconds, which is inadequate to ensure that the free mercury in the deeper aspects of the cavity rises through the considerable bulk of amalgam.

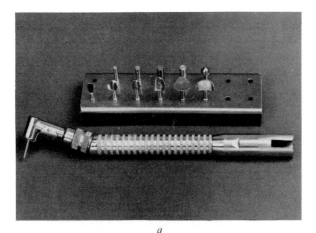

a

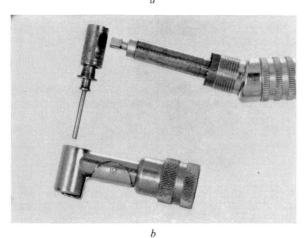

b

Fig. 93. *a*, Dentatus amalgam condenser with assortment of condensing points; *b*, Dismantled head of condenser showing how vibration is produced.

Ryge et al. (1952) have shown that better results will be obtained if the previously described technique is followed, that of using small increments of amalgam and condensing each with the small points, and removing excess plashy material before successive layers are added. When the cavity is overfilled, then the larger

89

points can be used. McHugh (1955) has also shown that successive small increments give better adaptation to the walls of the cavity.

Using the mechanical technique of condensation, dryer mixes of amalgam can be used, but care must be taken not to use the amalgam mixed after about 4 minutes from the time trituration was started, as the amalgam is beginning to crystallize and condensation will break up the crystalline form and lead to a weaker restoration.

Whatever the type of condensation technique used, it is essential to condense the amalgam into a space with rigid walls, and, if one of the walls yields during this process, crystallization is disturbed and weakness results. The need and methods for the correct and careful placing of a matrix in a two or more surfaced amalgam restoration, and also in larger Class V restorations, have been discussed. However, even with the most careful matrix placement and marginal adaptation, recent work with radioactive isotopes has changed our ideas of the degree of marginal adaptation attainable. Nelsen et al. (1952) and Sausen et al. (1953) have shown that no restorative material has perfect adaptation to the cavity walls. Nelsen et al. (1952) consider that the phenomenon of marginal percolation is due to the difference in the coefficient of expansion of the restoration, as compared with that of the tooth structure. However, Swartz and Phillips (1962) have shown that the marginal adaptation cannot really be related to expansion or contraction, as expanding or contracting amalgam restorations showed similar leakage patterns when using radioactive isotopes. Their work supported the fact that resistance to marginal leakage improved as the restoration aged, and that this initial leakage can be prevented by using a cavity varnish as a liner. This is supported by Barber et al. (1964) who have demonstrated the value of using a cavity varnish before inserting the amalgam restoration.

Leakage can be demonstrated with all restorations, although in a well-condensed amalgam restoration less has been observed. The reason given for the decrease in marginal leakage as the amalgam restoration ages is that the metallic ions and corrosive products slowly fill this space, and penetration of oral fluids is thereby prevented. It is also suggested that these ions may have some bacteriostatic effect. Cambell Smith (1949) mentions the oligodynamic properties of the metals, silver, tin, copper and zinc as being the cause of this bacteriostasis.

Although the exact clinical significance of marginal percolation with dyes and radioactive isotopes has not been established, it is interesting to note that from this aspect amalgam, provided it is properly inserted, is superior to all other commonly used restorative materials.

Finishing the Amalgam Restoration

Many flaws in amalgam restorations may be attributed to methods employed in finishing the restoration. Caries recurrence may occur in the stagnation areas formed by marginal excess of amalgam, or in the crevices resulting from the fracture of flakes or spur-like projections of amalgam at the periphery of the restoration. Schoonover and Souder (1941) have shown that even well-condensed amalgam fillings will corrode if they are not smooth at the margins and polished.

CARVING: From the foregoing it can be seen that it is essential to contour the restoration correctly by carving after the amalgam has been inserted into the cavity. As has been described in the condensing procedures, all amalgam fillings should be built to an excess, because the top portion is never as well condensed as the part underneath. Carving back to the desired anatomic form will then remove the

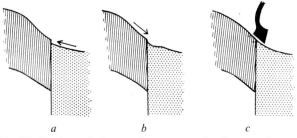

a   *b*   *c*

Fig. 94. Carving technique. *a,* Incorrect carving from amalgam to enamel; *b,* Incorrect carving from enamel to amalgam; *c,* Correct carving with blade of carving instrument resting on enamel and amalgam.

poorly condensed, mercury-rich amalgam, and leave thoroughly condensed amalgam with a satisfactory residual mercury content on the newly created surface of the finished restoration.

A sharp instrument should be used to cut amalgam, and the cutting should be done along the amalgam enamel junction, with part of the cutting blade resting on enamel (*Fig.* 94). This will help to obtain the correct occlusal anatomic form of the restoration. Carving should never be done in the direction of filling to enamel, because there is the risk of developing an enamel ledge by overcarving the amalgam (*Fig.* 94). Charbeneau (1965) and Kanai (1966) have shown the beneficial effect of burnishing the surface of the amalgam after carving. Svare and Chan (1972) did a study of the effect of surface treatment on the corrodibility of silver amalgam and showed that burnishing the amalgam surface after carving left it less likely to corrode than the unpolished carved surface or even the surface polished after 24 hours. There is certainly evidence to support the advantage of burnishing the amalgam surface immediately after carving and the previously held concept that this procedure has a deleterious effect on the amalgam surface does not appear to be supported.

A number of carving instruments have been developed, each in an attempt to provide a universal carver (*Fig*. 95). However, provided the blade is sharp and the design of the instrument allows the blade to follow the cavity outline while resting both on enamel and amalgam, it will serve as a useful instrument.

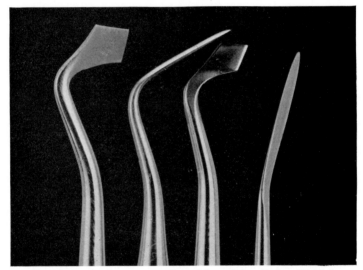

Fig. 95. Carving instruments. From left to right—Frahm, Ward 2, H, Ward 1.

A slight excess of amalgam should be left on all carved surfaces, except where it would cause occlusal interference, since carving leaves a rough surface, which can subsequently be polished away. It is essential that there is no occlusal interference, since this is probably the most common cause of fracture of amalgam restorations and post-restoration pain.

No attempt is made to reproduce deep anatomic fissures, as to do so can weaken the restoration, because of the reduced bulk of amalgam at the amalgam enamel junction. Mahler (1958) has shown that any surface discontinuities, such as carved developmental grooves, roughened surfaces, or inadvertent scratches or nicks, will produce harmful stress concentrations in an amalgam subjected to stresses. However, where the amalgam meets the enamel at a deep groove, such as a developmental groove, the amalgam must be carved to that groove, so as to ensure a smooth amalgam enamel junction.

Reference has already been made to Simon's suggested full bevel of enamel prisms, especially in high cusped teeth, where a cavo-surface line angle of 100° enhances the strength of the enamel. By not reproducing the natural depth of the fissure, the amalgam angle at the cavity margin can also be increased (*see Figs.* 36, 37). In this way both the enamel and amalgam margins are strengthened enormously. Hallett (1944), in supporting the concept of not fully reproducing the anatomic form when carving, suggests aiming to produce some degree of 'bas relief' in the amalgam, to simulate the anatomic form. In order to allow for this extra thickness of amalgam, it may be found necessary to adjust the occlusion by grinding the high points on the opposing cusps. In most cases this will not be necessary, since the opposing cusps rarely occlude with the deeper

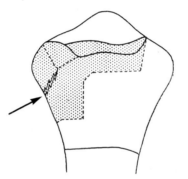

Fig. 96. Overcarving marginal ridge can lead to its subsequent fracture (arrow).

aspects of the fissures. Kantorowicz (1957) suggests carving a rounded fissure till the bite is just cleared of occlusal interference, so providing as strong an amalgam restoration as possible commensurate with not grinding an opposing cusp. Judicious limited grinding of an opposing enamel high point, however, is certainly justified, in order to produce a much more lasting and satisfactory amalgam restoration.

The marginal ridge, also, must not be excessively carved, as a narrow marginal ridge is easily fractured (*Fig.* 96). The marginal ridge should be wide and rounded, and the terminal fissures normally extending from the median fissure on to the occlusal inclined plane of the marginal ridge should be simulated. This will provide sluiceways to ensure the passage of food from the marginal ridge on to the occlusal surface and away from the interproximal areas.

The marginal ridge should, as a rule, be carved to the level of the adjacent marginal ridge; however, modifications may have to be made in cases of gross mal-relationship or malocclusion. The amalgam surface against the matrix should require no carving. If, however, there is any excess of amalgam at the buccal and lingual margins of the box, this should be carved away at this stage. Gross gingival excess should also be removed, and, in this regard, Miller (1952) is of the opinion that an X-ray should be taken at this stage, to see if there is any gingival overhang. The removal of a slight excess should be left until the final polishing of the amalgam restoration. Too often a broad, flat proximal surface is the result of instrumentation in carving proximal contours.

Castaldi et al. (1957) have shown that the use of dental floss as a means of contouring the proximal surface of the filling and removing gingival excess of amalgam is never as efficient as carefully contouring

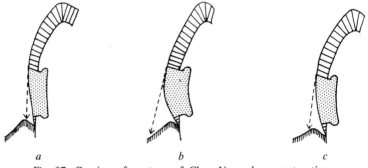

a   *b*   *c*

Fig. 97. Carving of contour of Class V amalgam restorations.
a, Undercontoured; *b*, Overcontoured; *c*, Correct contour.

the matrix band and wedging it in place. However, they have shown that, provided the flossing is done while the amalgam is still soft, there is some improvement of a poorly contoured proximal surface, and gingival excess can be removed. The dental floss should be passed between the teeth below the contact point, to avoid damage to the restoration in this area.

In Class V restorations it is necessary to contour the amalgam, in order to keep the gingival tissue healthy (*Fig.* 97). If the restoration is excessively bulged, the gingival tissues will not receive proper stimulation. On the other hand, if the restoration is insufficiently convex in contour, food will pass into the gingival crevice, with resultant gingival irritation. When carving a Class V amalgam restoration, slight excess of amalgam should be left, so that, after subsequent polishing procedures, the contour in the occlusogingival and mesiodistal directions will be correct.

POLISHING: Sweeney (1940) and Schoonover and Souder (1941) have shown that an amalgam restoration which has been highly polished is more resistant to corrosion and tarnish than one which is left unpolished. A tarnish layer usually forms on the polished surface, which tends to protect the amalgam, provided that it is uniformly distributed over the whole surface of the filling. Schoonover and Souder (1941) have stressed the importance of polishing the whole surface of the restoration, not only the easily accessible surface. They have shown that, if one portion of the restoration is not polished, it will tarnish to a greater extent than the polished surface; it then becomes a positive electrode in a voltaic cell, with the polished area being the negative electrode and the saliva forming the electrolyte. The polished area is thus corroded, and finally may become positive to the other area, which is corroded too, resulting in a cumulative process. This type of corrosion is particularly evident in areas where the cavity is not completely sealed by the filling; the products of this corrosion are carried into the dentinal tubules, with the resultant discoloration of the marginal area. This discoloration at the margins of an amalgam restoration has been called by Mosteller (1957) the 'amalgam line', and it is also seen in amalgam restorations where the enamel at the margin of the cavity is undermined, and the amalgam is, in fact, showing through. Mateer and Reitz (1970) have shown that the corrosion products formed on the surface of amalgam restorations consist mainly of the sulphides and oxides of tin.

Swartz et al. (1958) explain that the reason that completely unpolished amalgam restorations tarnish or corrode more easily than polished or partially polished restorations is because the surface roughness encourages the accumulation of food debris, which may contain sulphides. Unequal depositions on the surface encourage the formation of electric couples, and von Fraunhofer and Staheli (1971) have demonstrated the influence of plaque and calculus in affecting the formation of electric couples leading to corrosion.

Most authorities agree that polishing an amalgam restoration must be delayed for at least 24 hours, otherwise mercury, together with the weak tin-mercury phase, is brought to the surface. The weaker mercury-rich portions of the surface layer may be more easily removed during mastication, and thus leave a rough, pitted surface to the restoration.

One of the problems associated with silver amalgam is its relatively poor edge strength and its tendency to flow under stress. A cause of the ditched margin in well-finished amalgam restorations is due to the fact that the amalgam tends to creep up the cusp under normal masticatory stress. Subsequent fracture of this weak spur of amalgam will produce this ditched margin (*Fig.* 98) which provides an excellent nidus for recurrent caries. Matsuda and Fusayama (1970) in their experiments, support this need to service amalgam restorations regularly especially after the first six months, by grinding away rough edges and so produce a smooth amalgam enamel junction.

In producing a smooth, occlusal surface to the amalgam restoration, Grundy (1959) has shown that good results are obtained with a

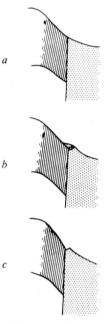

Fig. 98. Effect of marginal creep of amalgam leading from *a*, smooth amalgam-enamel junction; *b*, turned edge of amalgam on enamel resulting from marginal flow; *c*, ditched margin resulting from fracture of turned edge.

well-worn or blunted finishing burr, followed by polishing with whitening in alcohol applied with a bristle brush. The blunted finishing burr will adequately remove marginal excesses of amalgam, and also make modifications to the anatomic form of the restoration. However, should gross occlusal excesses of amalgam be present, these can more easily be removed with carborundum stones before smoothing with the finishing burr.

Fine sandpaper discs can be used to polish the buccal and lingual embrasures of proximal surfaces, the proximal amalgam above the contact area, Class V restorations, and the buccal and lingual extensions from occlusal restorations.

The proximal amalgam below the contact area is polished with linen strips after removing any gingival excess of amalgam with amalgam files (*Fig.* 99). Gingival excess of amalgam should not be removed with a revolving burr since this can cause trauma to the gingival tissue and to the adjacent tooth or restoration. The E.V.A. Prophylaxis System (*Fig.* 100) is a very useful tool in this situation when the safe-sided and safe-edged diamond tip is used. The tip is fitted into a piston in the head of the handpiece which is oscillated by an eccentric cam driven by the dental engine. The diamond tip consequently has a reciprocal action and, with a stroke of 1·5 mm, results

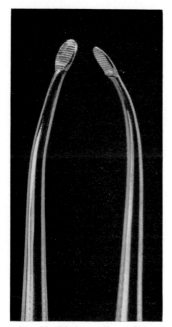

Fig. 99. Rhein amalgam files.

in a scrubbing effect when placed against the amalgam. Ultrasonic scaler points are also useful in removing gingival excess of amalgam. The contact area itself should not be polished for fear of opening up the contact point. It is for this reason that a smooth, highly polished matrix band is used, in order to ensure that the smoothest possible surface of amalgam is left in contact with the adjacent tooth.

The final polishing to produce a high lustre is achieved with tin oxide or whitening made into a paste with alcohol and applied to the tooth with a bristle brush. Grundy (1959) advises against using a rubber cup, as it tends to work up wave-like mounds in the amalgam, and Kantorowicz (1957) recommends a goat-hair brush in preference to a bristle or nylon brush. Care should be taken when polishing not to raise the surface temperature too high. Mitchell et al. (1955) have warned that when polishing techniques produce temperatures above 65° C mercury is

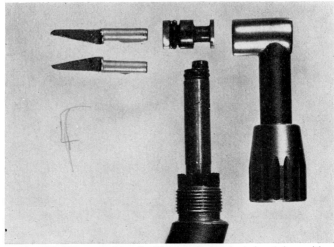

Fig. 100. Dismantled head of E.V.A. Prophylaxis handpiece with right and left safe-sided diamond tips.

released from the amalgam, which will result in weakened or defective areas in the restoration, and there is the additional risk of pulpal injury. The use of alcohol to form a paste, and a technique of intermittently applying the polishing brush, will ensure that the surface temperature of the amalgam does not become too high.

REFERENCES

Acharya A., Sarkar N. K., Marker B. D. and Greener E. H. (1973) Some physical properties of an admixed high copper amalgam. *J. Dent. Res.* **52**, 187.

Ambrose E. R. (1962) Pressure amalgamation. *J. Can. Dent. Assoc.* **28**, 571.

Amler M. H. (1948) Radioactive phosphate permeability in dentin following the use of medicaments. *J. Dent. Res.* **27**, 635.

App G. R. (1961) The effect of silicate, amalgam and cast gold on the gingiva. *J. Prosthet. Dent.* **11**, 522.

Baker D. L. and Curson I. (1974) A high speed method for finishing cavity margins. *Br. Dent. J.* **137**, 391.

Baldwin H. (1897) Cement and amalgam fillings. *Trans. Odontol. Soc. Lond.* 2nd ser., **29**, 93.

Barber D., Lyell J. and Massler M. (1964) Effectiveness of copal resin varnish under amalgam restorations. *J. Prosthet. Dent.* **14**, 533.

Basker R. M., Spence D. and Wilson H. J. (1973) The strength of amalgam. A comparative study of test methods using various alloys. *Br. Dent. J.* **135**, 369.

Basker R. M. and Wilson H. J. (1971) Spherical particle amalgam. *Br. Dent. J.*, **130**, 338.

Batt H. (1942) Gibt es ein Kariesrezidiv? *Schweiz. Monatsschr. Zahnheilkd.* **52**, 753.

Berman D. S. (1958) Pulpal healing following experimental pulpotomy. *Br. Dent. J.* **105**, 7.

Besic F. C. (1943) The fate of bacteria sealed in dental cavities. *J. Dent. Res.* **22**, 349.

Black G. V. (1947) *Operative Dentistry*, 8th ed. Chicago, Medico-Dental Publishing Co.

Blackwell R. E. (1940) A consideration of the location of the gingival margin in cavity preparation. *NorthWest. Univ. Bull.* **41**, No. 1, 4.

Boyde A. (1973) Finishing techniques for the exit margin of the approximal portion of Class II cavities. *Br. Dent. J.*, **134**, 319.

Boyde A. and Knight P. J. (1972) Scanning electron microscope studies of Class II cavity margins: matrix band application. *Br. Dent. J.* **133**, 331.

Boyde A., Knight P. J. and Jones S. J. (1972) Further scanning electron microscope studies of the preparation of Class II cavities. *Br. Dent. J.* **132**, 447.

Braden M. (1964) Heat conduction in teeth and the effect of lining materials. *J. Dent. Res.* **43**, 315.

Bronner F. J. (1931) Mechanical, physiological, and pathological aspects of operative procedures. *Dent. Cosmos* **73**, 577.

Brown G. (1955) Matrices for deciduous teeth. *Dent. Pract. Dent. Rec.* **6**, 78.

Bull F. A. (1936) A simple method of improving amalgam restorations. *J. Am. Dent. Assoc.* **23**, 1880.

Castaldi C., Phillips R. W. and Clark R. J. (1957) Further studies on the contour of Class II restorations with various matrix technics. *J. Dent. Res.* **36**, 462.

Chan K. C. and Svare C. W. (1972) Mercury vapor emission from dental amalgam. *J. Dent. Res.* **51**, 555.

Charbeneau G. T. (1965) A suggested technique for polishing amalgam restorations. *J. Mich. Dent. Assoc.* **47**, 320.

Cook T. A. and Yates P. O. (1969) Fatal mercury intoxication in a dental surgery assistant. *Br. Dent. J.* **127**, 553.

Crowell W. S. and Phillips R. W. (1951) Physical properties of amalgam as influenced by variation in surface area of the alloy particles. *J. Dent. Res.* **30**, 845.

De Boer J. G. (1956) Dental caries: operative and restorative therapy. *Int. Dent. J.* **6**, 401.

Demajo A. P. (1954) Placement of the gingival margin in proximal cavity preparation. *Dent. Surv.* **30**, 1551.

Demaree N. C. and Taylor D. F. (1962) Properties of dental amalgams made from spherical alloy particles. *J. Dent. Res.* **41**, 890.

Dilts W. E., Welk D. A. and Stovall J. (1968) Retentive properties of pin materials in pin-retained silver amalgam restorations. *J. Am. Dent. Assoc.* **77**, 1085.

Duperon D. F. and Kasloff Z. (1971) Effects of three types of pins on compressive strength of dental amalgam. *J. Can. Dent. Assoc.* **37**, 422.

Eames W. B. (1959) Preparation and condensation of amalgam with a low mercury alloy ratio. *J. Am. Dent. Assoc.* **58**, 78.

Eames W. B., Skinner E. W. and Mizera G. T. (1961) Amalgam strength values relative to mercury percentages and plasticity. *J. Prosthet. Dent.* **11**, 765.

Ferrier W. I. (1959) *Gold Foil Operations.* Seattle, University of Washington Press.

Fisher F. J. (1969) The viability of micro-organisms in carious dentine beneath amalgam restorations. An appendix. *Br. Dent. J.* **126**, 355.

Fisher, F. J. (1972) The effect of a calcium hydroxide water paste on micro-organisms in carious dentine. *Br. Dent. J.* **133**, 19.

Forsten L. (1969) Physical properties of dental amalgams. A study of standard and preamalgamated zinc-containing and zinc-free amalgams uncontaminated and contaminated with moisture. Academic dissertation, University of Turku, Turku, Finland.

Fraunhofer J. A. von and Staheli P. J. (1971) Corrosion of amalgam restorations: a new explanation. *Br. Dent. J.* **130**, 522.

Fraunhofer J. A. von and Staheli P. J. (1972) Gold-amalgam galvanic cells. The measurement of corrosion currents. *Br. Dent. J.* **132**, 357.

Frykholm K. O. (1957) On mercury from dental amalgam: its toxic and allergic effects and some comments on occupational hygiene. *Acta Odontol. Scand.* **15**, Suppl. 22.

Gabel A. B. (1954) *American Textbook of Operative Dentistry*, 9th ed. London, Kimpton.

Gabel A. B. (1957) Present day concepts of cavity preparation. *Dent. Clin. North Am.* **3**, March.

REFERENCES

Gayler Marie L. V. (1934) Some factors affecting the setting of a dental amalgam, Pt II. *Br. Dent. J.* **56**, 605.

Going R. E. (1966) Pin-retained amalgam. *J. Am. Dent. Assoc.* **73**, 619.

Going R. E. and Massler M. (1961) Influence of cavity liners under amalgam restorations on penetration by radioactive isotopes. *J. Prosthet. Dent.* **11**, 298.

Going R. E., Massler M. and Dute H. L. (1960) Marginal penetration of dental restorations by different radioactive isotopes. *J. Dent. Res.* **39**, 273.

Goldstein P. M. (1966) Retention pins are friction-locked without use of cement. *J. Am. Dent. Assoc.* **73**, 1103.

Granath L.-E. and Möller B. (1971) Reaction of the human dental pulp to silver amalgam restorations. Effect of insertion of amalgam of high plasticity in shallow cavities. *Acta Odontol. Scand.* **29**, 165.

Gray A. W. (1919) Metallographic phenomena observed in amalgams. *J. Natl Dent. Assoc.* **6**, 513 ad 909.

Green R. O., Shellman J. F. and Simon W. J. (1943) Manipulation of amalgam. *J. Am. Dent. Assoc.* **30**, 1168.

Grundy J. R. (1959) The effects of abrasive agents on an amalgam surface. *Dent. Pract. Dent. Rec.* **9**, 262.

Guard W. F., Haack D. C. and Ireland R. L. (1958) Photo-elastic stress analysis of bucco-lingual sections of Class II Cavity restorations. *J. Am. Dent. Assoc.* **57**, 631.

Hallett G. E. M. (1944) Amalgam restorations in fissural cavities in posterior teeth. *Br. Dent. J.* **76**, 4.

Harvey W. (1946) Some recent research into dental amalgams at the R.A.F. Institute of Aviation Medicine, Farnborough, Hants. *Br. Dent. J.* **81**, 245.

Hatt S. D. (1959) The relationship of amalgam to the cavity wall. *Dent. Pract. Dent. Rec.* **10**, 76.

Healey H. J. and Phillips R. W. (1949) A clinical study of amalgam failures. *J. Dent. Res.* **28**, 439.

Hitchin A. D. and Hall D. C. (1963) Allergic lesions of the tongue due to silver content of amalgam fillings. *Dent. Pract. Dent. Rec.* **14**, 143.

Hoppenstand D. C. and McConnell D. (1960) Mechanical failures of amalgam restorations with zinc phosphate and zinc oxide/eugenol cement bases. *J. Dent. Res.* **39**, 899.

Innes D. B. K. and Youdelis W. V. (1963) Dispersion strengthened amalgams. *J. Canad. Dent. Assoc.* **29**, 587.

Jarabak J. R. (1942) The effect of particle size on dimensional change in dental amalgams. *J. Am. Dent. Assoc.* **29**, 593.

Jerman A. C. (1970) Silver amalgam restorative material with stannous fluoride. *J. Am. Dent. Assoc.* **80**, 787.

Jørgensen K. D., Esbensen A. L. and Borring-Møller G. (1966) The effect of porosity and mercury content upon the strength of silver amalgam. *Acta Odontol. Scand.* **24**, 535.

Jørgensen K. D., Holst K. and Palbøl O. P. (1964) Mercury content of silver amalgam. Influence of time between completion of the mix and start of condensation. *Acta Odontol. Scand.* **22**, 207.

Jordan R. E. and Suzuki M. (1971) Conservative treatment of deep carious lesions. *J. Can. Dent. Assoc.* **37**, 337.

Kanai S. (1966) Effect of burnishing on the margins of occlusal amalgam restorations. *J. Japan Res. Soc. Dent. Mat. Appl.* **13**, 16 March.

Kantorowicz G. F. (1957) Finishing amalgam restorations. *Dent. Pract. Dent. Rec.* **8**, 64.

Karlström S. (1950) Amalgam condensing by means of ultra sounds. *Sven. Tandlak. Tidskr.* **43**, 297.

Koran A. and Asgar K. (1967) A comparison of dental amalgams made from a spherical alloy and from a comminuted alloy. *J. Am. Dent. Assoc.* **75**, 912.

Kornfield B. (1952) Amalgam restorations, in *Handbook of Dental Practice* (ed. Grossman), 2nd ed. London, New Era Publishing Co.

Kraus A. (1945) From engineering to physiology. *Br. Dent. J.* **78**, 230.

Kraus A. (1952) Considérations sur les bases scientifiques des méthodes de traitement actuelles des dents cariées. *Schweiz. Monatsschr. Zahnheilkd.* **62**, 1232.

Link W. A. (1944) Anatomic amalgam restorations. *J. Am. Dent. Assoc.* **31**, 1211.

Lyell J. S. (1960) Base forming materials for restorations of silver amalgam. *Aust. Dent. J.* **5**, 132.

McCall J. O. (1926) Studies in the etiology of approximal and gingival caries. *J. Dent. Res.* **6**, 461.

MacDonald R. E. and Phillips R. W. (1950) Clinical observations on a contracting amalgam alloy. *J. Dent. Res.* **29**, 482.

McGehee W. H. O., True H. A. and Inskipp E. F. (1956) *A Textbook of Operative Dentistry*, 4th ed. New York, McGraw-Hill.

McHugh W. D. (1955) Experiments on the hardness and adaptation of dental amalgam as affected by various condensation techniques. *Br. Dent. J.* **99**, 44.

Mahler D. B. (1958) An analysis of stresses in a dental amalgam restoration. *J. Dent. Res.* **37**, 516.

Mahler D. B. and Armen G. K. (1962) Addition of amalgam alloy to zinc-phosphate cement. *J. Prosthet. Dent.* **12**, 157.

Mahler D. B., Terkla L. G. and Van Eysden J. (1973) Marginal fracture of amalgam restorations. *J. Dent. Res.* **52**, 823.

Markley M. R. (1951) Restorations of silver amalgam. *J. Am. Dent. Assoc.* **43**, 133.

Markley M. R. (1955) Amalgam restorations for Class V cavities. *J. Am. Dent. Assoc.* **50**, 301.

Markley M. R. (1958) Pin reinforcement and retention of amalgam foundations and restorations, *J. Am. Dent. Assoc.* **56**, 675.

Mateer R. S. and Reitz C. D. (1970) Corrosion of amalgam restorations. *J. Dent. Res.* **49**, 399.

Matsuda N. and Fusayama T. (1970) Marginal fracture of amalgam restorations. *J. Prosthet. Dent.* **23**, 658.

Miller E. C. (1952) Construction of the amalgam restoration. *J. Can. Dent. Assoc.* **18**, 119.

REFERENCES

Mitchell J. A., Dickson G. and Schoonover I. C. (1955) X-ray diffraction studies of mercury diffusion and surface stability of dental amalgam. *J. Dent. Res.* **34**, 744.

Mizera G. T. and Skinner E. W. (1961) Effect of amalgam condensation on compressive strength. *J. Dent. Res.* **40**, 771.

Moffa J. P., Razzano M. R. and Doyle M. G. (1969) Pins—a comparison of their retentive properties. *J. Am. Dent. Assoc.* **78**, 529.

Möller B. and Granath L.-E. (1973) Reaction of the human dental pulp to silver amalgam restorations. The effect of insertion of amalgam of high plasticity in deep cavities. *Acta Odontol. Scand.* **31**, 187.

Moss R. P., jun. (1953) Amalgam failures. *U.S. Armed Fcs Med. J.* **4**, 735.

Mosteller J. H. (1950) Principles of condensation of amalgam. *J. Georgia Dent. Assoc.* **24**, 10.

Mosteller J. H. (1957) Role of silver amalgam in a modern dental practice. *J. Am. Dent. Assoc.* **55**, 335.

Nadal R., Phillips R. W. and Swartz M. L. (1961) Clinical investigation on the relation of mercury to the amalgam restoration. *J. Am. Dent. Assoc.* **63**, 8 and 488.

Nakamura T., Fischer T. E., Habu H. and Nagai K. (1961) Amalgam properties when mixed by pressure only. *J. Dent. Res.* **40**, 772.

Nelsen R. J., Wolcott R. B. and Paffenbarger G. C. (1952) Fluid exchange at the margins of dental restorations. *J. Am. Dent. Assoc.* **44**, 288.

Nicholls E. (1963) The restoration of root filled teeth. *Dent. Prac. Dent. Rec.* **13**, 459.

Nixon G. S. and Rowbotham T. C. (1971) Mercury hazards associated with high speed mechanical amalgamators. *Br. Dent. J.* **131**, 308.

Pearson S. L. (1959) Better amalgam fillings. *Dent. Pract. Dent. Rec.*, **9**, 208.

Petersen E. A. and Freedman G. (1972) Laminate reinforced dental amalgam. *J. Dent. Res.* **51**, 79.

Peyton F. A., Anthony D. H., Asgar K., Charbeneau G. T., Craig R. G. and Myers G. E. (1960) *Restorative Dental Materials.* St. Louis, C. V. Mosby.

Phillips L. J., Phillips R. W. and Schnell R. J. (1955) Measurement of the electric conductivity of dental cement. IV. Extracted human teeth: in vivo tests; Summary. *J. Dent. Res.* **34**, 839.

Phillips R. W. (1944) Physical properties of amalgam as influenced by the mechanical amalgamator and pneumatic condenser. *J. Am. Dent. Assoc.* **31**, 1308.

Phillips R. W. (1963) Report of the Committee on Scientific Investigations of the American Academy of Restorative Dentistry. *J. Prosthet. Dent.* **13**, 515.

Phillips R. W. (1973) Selection of amalgam alloys: particle form, new formulas. *J. Dent. Child.* **40**, 106.

Phillips R. W. and Boyd D. A. (1947) Importance of the mercury alloy ratio to the amalgam filling. *J. Am. Dent. Assoc.* **34**, 451.

Phillips R. W., Boyd D. A., Healey H. J. and Crawford W. H. (1945) Clinical observations on amalgam with known physical properties—Final Report. *J. Am. Dent. Assoc.* **32**, 324.

Phillips R. W., Castaldi C. R., Rinard J. R. and Clark R. J. (1956) Proximal contour of Class II amalgam restorations made with various matrix band technics. *J. Am. Dent. Assoc.* **53**, 391.

Phillips R. W. and Swartz M. L. (1949) Mercury analysis of one hundred amalgam restorations. *J. Dent. Res.* **28**, 569.

Phillips R. W., Swartz M. L. and Boozayaangool R. (1954) Effect of moisture contamination on the compressive strength of amalgam. *J. Am. Dent. Assoc.* **49**, 436.

Pickard H. M. (1973) *A Manual of Operative Dentistry*, 3rd ed. London, Oxford University Press.

Plant C. G. (1970) The effect of polycarboxylate cement on the dental pulp: a study. *Br. Dent. J.* **129**, 424.

Plant C. G. and Wilson H. J. (1970) Early strengths of lining materials. *Br. Dent. J.* **129**, 269.

Plant C. G. and Wilson H. J. (1971). Forces exerted on lining materials. *Br. Dent. J.* **131**, 62.

Ramsay K. P. (1941) A rational technic for amalgam restorations. *J. Am. Dent. Assoc.* **28**, 523.

Romnes A. F. (1953) Amalgam restorations: a critical survey of present-day practice. *Int. Dent. J.* **4**, 1.

Roper L. H. (1947) Restorations with amalgam in the army: An evaluation and analysis. *J. Am. Dent. Assoc.* **34**, 443.

Ryge G., Dickson G., Smith D. L. and Schoonover I. C. (1952) Dental amalgam: the effect of mechanical condensation on some physical properties. *J. Am. Dent. Assoc.* **45**, 269.

Ryge G., Fairhurst C. W. and Oberbreckling R. E. (1958) Proportion of dental amalgam. *J. Am. Dent. Assoc.* **57**, 496.

Sausen R. E., Armstrong W. D. and Simon W. J. (1953) Penetration of radio-calcium at margin of acrylic restorations made by compression and non-compression technics. *J. Am. Dent. Assoc.* **47**, 636.

Schoonover I. C. and Souder W. (1941) Corrosion of dental alloys. *J. Am. Dent. Assoc.* **28**, 1278.

Shovelton D. S. (1968) Silver amalgam and mercury allergy. *Oral Surg.* **25**, 29.

Shovelton D. S. (1972) The maintenance of pulp vitality. *Br. Dent. J.* **133**, 95.

Simon W. J. (1951) Fundamental differences between the amalgam and the inlay cavity preparation. *J. Am. Dent. Assoc.* **42**, 307.

Simon W. J. (ed.) (1956) *Clinical Operative Dentistry*. Philadelphia, Saunders.

Skinner E. W. and Phillips R. W. (1960) *The Science of Dental Materials*, 5th ed. Philadelphia, Saunders.

Smith D. C. (1968) A new dental cement. *Br. Dent. J.* **125**, 381.

Smith J. Cambell (1949) *The Chemistry and Metallurgy of Dental Materials*, 2nd ed. Oxford, Blackwell.

Staheli P. J. and Fraunhofer J. A. von (1971) Micro-hardness. Micro-hardness and compressive strength of preamalgamated and non-preamalgamated conventional and spherical amalgam alloys: a comparative study. *Br. Dent. J.* **131**, 145.

REFERENCES

Stoner G. E., Senti S. E. and Gileadi E. (1971) Effect of sodium flouride and stannous flouride on the rate of corrosion of dental amalgams. *J. Dent. Res.* **50**, 1647.

Svare C. W. and Chan K. C. (1972) Effect of surface treatment on corrodibility of dental amalgam. *J. Dent. Res.* **51**, 44.

Swartz M. L. and Phillips R. W. (1956) Residual mercury content of amalgam restorations and its influence on compressive strength. *J. Dent. Res.* **35**, 458.

Swartz M. L. and Phillips R. W. (1961) In vitro studies on the marginal leakage of restorative materials. *J. Am. Dent. Assoc.* **62**, 141.

Swartz M. L. and Phillips R. W. (1962) Influence of manipulative variables on the marginal adaptation of certain restorative materials. *J. Prosthet. Dent.* **12**, 172.

Swartz M. L., Phillips R. W. and El Tannir M. D. (1958) Tarnish of certain dental alloys. *J. Dent. Res.* **37**, 837.

Sweeney J. T. (1940) Amalgam manipulation: manual *v.* mechanical aids, Part II—Comparison of clinical applications. *J. Am. Dent. Assoc.* **27**, 1940.

Sweeney J. T. (1941) Delayed expansion in non-zinc alloys. *J. Am. Dent. Assoc.* **28**, 2018.

Sweeney J. T. (1944) Manipulation of amalgam to prevent excessive distortion and corrosion. *J. Am. Dent. Assoc.* **31**, 375.

Swerdlow H. and Stanley H. R. (1962) Response of the human dental pulp to amalgam restorations. *Oral Surg.* **15**, 499.

Thanik K. D., Boyd D. A. and Van Huysen G. (1962) Cavity base materials and the exposed pulp marginal blood-vessels. *J. Prosthet. Dent.* **12**, 165.

Vale W. A. (1959) Cavity preparation and further thoughts on high speed. *Br. Dent. J.* **107**, 333.

Van Gunst I. C. A. and Hertog H. J. P. M. (1957) On the relation between delayed expansion of amalgam and the composition of amalgam alloys. *Br. Dent. J.* **103**, 428.

Waerhaug J. (1960) Histologic considerations which govern where the margins of restorations should be located in relation to the gingiva. *Dent. Clin. North Am.* **161**, March.

Walter M. (1960) Pin reinforcement for amalgam restorations. *Br. Dent. J.* **108**, 194.

Welk D. A. and Dilts W. E. (1967) Influence of pins on the compressive and transverse strength of dental amalgam and retention of pins in amalgam. *J. Am. Dent. Assoc.* **78**, 101.

Wing G. (1965) Pin retention amalgam restorations. *Aust. Dent. J.* **10**, 6.

Wing G. (1966) Spherical particle amalgams. *Aust. Dent. J.* **11**, 265.

Zander H. A. (1940) Bacteria in the dentin after cavity preparation. *Illinois Dent. J.* **9**, 207.

Zander H. A. (1954) The treatment of dentine before insertion of restorations. *Int. Dent. J.* **4**, 693.

Zander H. A. (1957) Effect of silicate cement and amalgam on the gingiva. *J. Am. Dent. Assoc.* **55**, 11.

INDEX